THE EVERYDAY
Heart-Healthy
COOKBOOK

THE EVERYDAY
Heart-Healthy
COOKBOOK

75 Gluten-Free, Dairy-Free, Clean Food Recipes

Breeana Pooler

Foreword by James LaValle, America's wellness expert

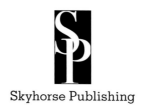

Skyhorse Publishing

Skyhorse Publishing books may be purchased in bulk at special discounts for sales promotion, corporate gifts, fund-raising, or educational purposes. Special editions can also be created to specifications. For details, contact the Special Sales Department, Skyhorse Publishing, 307 West 36th Street, 11th Floor, New York, NY 10018 or info@skyhorsepublishing.com.

Skyhorse® and Skyhorse Publishing® are registered trademarks of Skyhorse Publishing, Inc.®, a Delaware corporation.

Visit our website at www.skyhorsepublishing.com.

10 9 8 7 6 5 4 3 2 1

Library of Congress Cataloging-in-Publication Data is available on file.

Cover design by Daniel Brount

Print ISBN: 978-1-5107-6477-4
Ebook ISBN: 978-1-5107-6684-6

Printed in China

"Cooking is one of those great gifts you can give to those you love." —Ina Garten

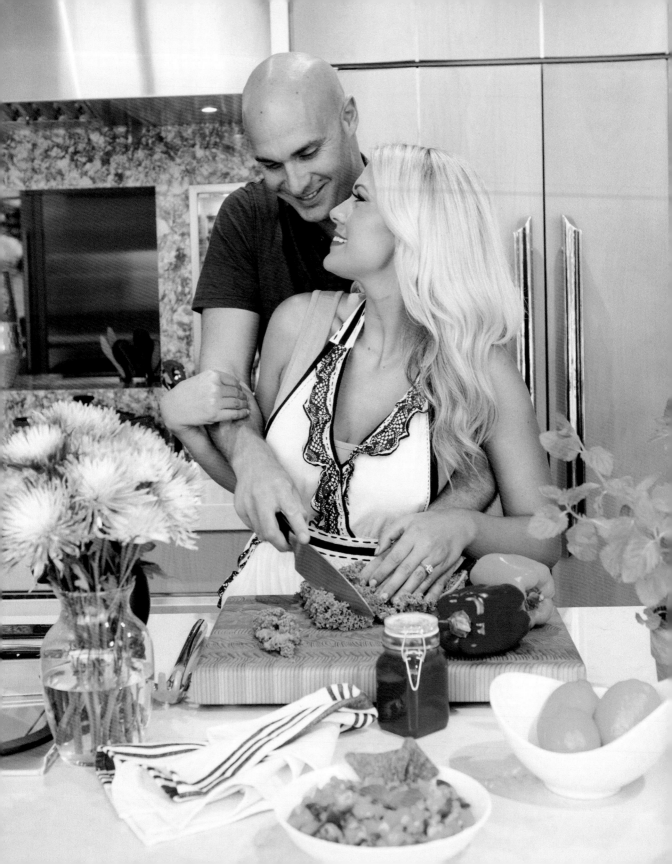

Contents

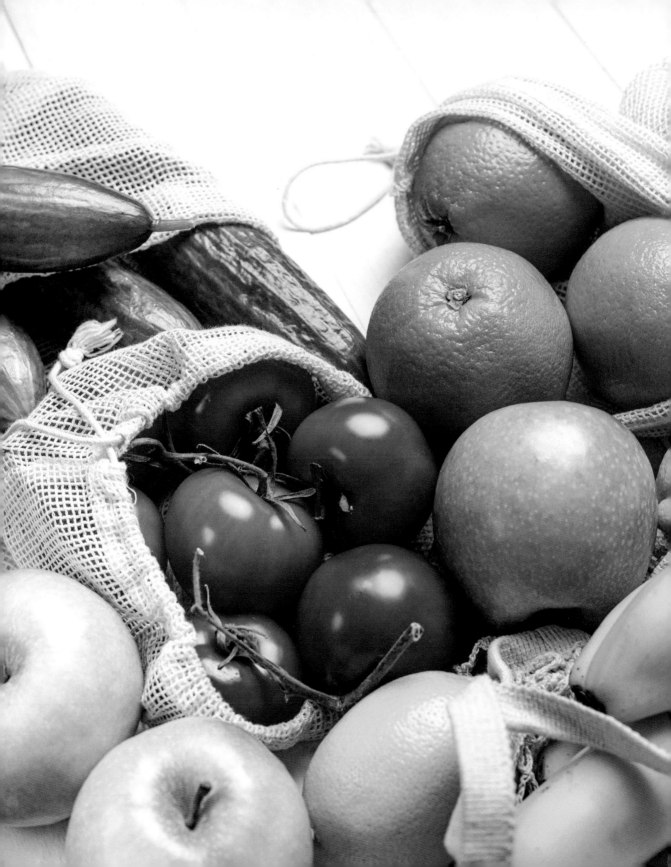

Foreword

By James LaValle, America's Wellness Expert, Clinical Pharmacist, Board Certified Clinical Nutritionist

A few years ago, I had a client referred to me—I must say it was one of the more heart-wrenching cases I've had over the years. A young man, just newly wed, walked in with a defibrillator vest on and told me his heart had gone into failure. It was medically classified as an idiopathic (unknown cause) cardiomyopathy. Though he survived, he remained very weak and unable to resume normal activity months out from the event. His color was ashen, and I knew we would have some work ahead, but I felt fairly confident we could at least get him some improvement.

Naturally, his family members were also stunned by the event and were very concerned for his prognosis. What sort of future would he have when he could barely perform normal daily activities, much less his former active life? Perplexing as it was, he had just played several hours of basketball a few days before this event. His cardiologist said not to expect an improvement in something called ejection fraction (a measurement of how much blood leaves the heart with each beat), which at that point was very low. He was also told he would most likely be put on a transplant list if certain heart functions did not improve.

So, I got to work using what we in integrative health practices call a "systems biology assessment approach," to determine which systems or networks in his body needed the most support. This particularly includes: the patient's history since birth, drugs they'd been on, illnesses they've had, how they slept, what their stress levels were like, diet, etc. In other words, we really try to get an understanding of how he ended up in the health crisis he was suffering—what underlying health issues could have possibly contributed to the heart failure of a man *so young*.

Then, we assess what nutrients and other nutritional supplements we could use to help correct underlying issues, while also supporting the heart itself to restore his health as much as possible. I found the primary area in need of support was his gut health. In physically assessing Jason, one of the things that stood out was the presence of soft white patches in the skin, which I recognized as a fungal skin condition and which are often overlooked in conventional medical care as just some sort of idiopathic skin pigmentation issue. Upon inquiring, I found out he'd had it since his teenage years. Jason's event actually occurred just about the same time that medical research began linking something called lipopolysaccharides and heart failure. Lipopolysaccharides are toxic substances from dying gut bacteria that can leak into the bloodstream and cause damage to the heart muscle. It's a long story, but a true one, and by addressing that issue, along with the use of certain key nutrients (like CoQ10, carnitine, taurine, and creatine pyruvate) which are supportive for the function of heart muscle tissue, Jason did start to—over time—regain strength and resiliency, and is now living very actively and normally once again. It was exciting the first time he could walk into my office and not have that defibrillator vest on anymore!

What went into his recovery program? I have spent the last thirty-three years of my life researching the use of dietary supplements as supportive treatment for people in chronic conditions. Jason still needed his cardiologist, and he still needed to be on the medications he was on, but he was stuck and not improving. Diet and targeted nutrients could help his body get the inertia needed to rejuvenate his health—even if we only got partway there, it beat being stuck where he was.

First, we used dietary supplements to replete and restore nutrients or address other issues that were important to his condition.

For the most part, I selected nutrients to support his heart, but sprinkled in some supplements for his gut health as well.

For Jason's heart:

- CoQ10 is a molecule in the body that helps produce energy in the cells needed for all cell functions. It is also an antioxidant. It has helped people in heart failure improve their ejection fraction and it has been published in studies, so it was a no-brainer first step.
- Adding l-carnitine (an amino acid that is naturally produced in the body and plays a role in helping with energy production for cells) helps with improving ability to exercise, peak oxygen capacity, and has been shown to improve ejection fraction by as much as 13.6 percent. Anything that helps energy production in the body is especially important for the heart.
- D-Ribose—this is a sugar found in the B vitamin riboflavin, that is a fuel source for the muscle (heart muscles in particular) and can improve ventricle efficiency. That was important because we didn't want Jason's heart to overwork and enlarge any more. Multiple studies have reported that ribose helps to restore energy production in the heart after an event like Jason's.

- Creatine Pyruvate (creatine that has been bound with pyruvic acid) has been used for performance enhancement for a few years, but it made sense to select this supportive nutrient for Jason. In several trials, creatine had shown the ability to improve difficulty breathing under physical exertion. One of my goals for Jason was to be able to exercise again and maybe even get back on the basketball court.
- Taurine—this amino acid, important for cardiac muscle energetics, was added because two studies showed that this amino acid could improve ejection fraction and exercise capacity in as little as two weeks.
- Magnesium is a key mineral that is essential to efficient muscular contraction and since Jason had previously had a major sweet tooth, his diet was very poor in minerals like this. Low magnesium has been linked to all sorts of cardiometabolic problems. In addition, I wanted to include this nutrient because one of the meds he was on is known to deplete magnesium.
- Nicotinamide Riboside/PQQ—both of these nutraceuticals help with mitochondrial rejuvenation, or in other words, help the powerhouses of the muscles. While this effects all muscle tissue, again I was primarily concerned with support for the heart muscle specifically.
- Vector 450 was used. This is an egg-based immunoglobulin we used to help strengthen Jason's immunity, in case a virus had been involved in the heart failure.

For his gut health:

I believe this was as important an aspect to Jason's program as anything that we did. A great deal of research has come out in the past decade regarding the role of lipo-polysaccharide (LPS). This is the byproduct of poor blood perfusion to the gut, which leads to the die off of the flora in the intestine. When flora die off they send LPS molecules all over the body, attaching to various muscle tissue, including the heart, triggering damage to those tissues. He had all that fungus in his skin. The primary source of systemic fungus is from the gut. What shows up on the outside started on the inside. We used gut restorative supplements like probiotics and cat's claw, berberine, and caprylic acid to rebalance gut flora along with things like specialty aloe vera extracts that help rebuild gut linings. We were trying to prevent further damage to the heart by healing the gut. Worsening of heart failure has recently been postulated to be the result of this LPS activity.

For his diet:

The next component of healing was to address the quality of his diet. First, when gut permeability is an issue, a key dietary measure is to consume a low-allergen diet. Because the immune system in the gut can create inflammatory chemicals in response to allergenic proteins in food, we recommended a diet that was wheat- and gluten-free, and dairy-free (wheat and cow's milk contain the most allergenic proteins of any foods).

Secondly, we recommended a very low-sugar diet. Jason had a real sweet tooth. Sugar can contribute to imbalances in gut flora and make one more prone to the effects of pathogenic bacteria like E. coli. In addition, it can deplete important nutrients like chromium and B-vitamins.

These were my primary concerns, however, I also wanted to teach Jason how to eat to prevent any problems in the future. We wanted to help prevent insulin resistance and diabetes for his future heart health, so having a lower intake of high glycemic foods was important. In addition, other anti-inflammatory dietary measures include eating a lot of vegetables and moderate intake of fruits that are high in antioxidants and other phytochemicals that protect our health, while making sure to take in plenty of omega-3 fats.

Finally, a key component of diet in most integrative practitioners' books is to eat as chemically-free as possible. This means eating foods that have not been grown with chemical pesticides, or in the case of animal proteins, that have been fed foods treated with pesticides. Whether it is choosing to buy foods that are sustainably raised or that have the USDA Organic label, we look at this as an important measure because food chemicals have now been found to be metabolically disruptive, affecting immunity, thyroid hormones, and insulin resistance, just to name a few effects.

The bottom line is that it is no longer a question "if" chemicals used in growing food can affect human health, it is known for sure that they do, and the effects are probably more far-reaching than most people would ever believe. Therefore, in an effort to eat as health consciously as possible, it makes sense that lowered intake of disruptive chemicals would be helpful.

Taking this a step further, one may want to try to limit other exposures. Environmental exposures to other toxins like lead have also been cited as having an effect directly on heart function. Lead is one of the heavy metals that can be very disruptive to health. It can cause high blood pressure and it can contribute to osteoporosis, for example, not to mention the learning issues it can cause in children. To help avoid exposure, you can have your tap water tested for lead levels. I have always believed you need to be empowered to know how to live in the ecoculture we currently are in, and the more proactive you can be in lowering these types of exposures, the more you can lower risks and the healthier you can be.

The above measures were my recommendations for Jason. I make "recommendations" for people every day and teach health-care professionals how to create individual programs such as the one I gave Jason. However, it is not what gets recommended that improves one's health, but if the person actually abides by those recommendations when they get home. I must say in this area, Breeana and Jason were rock stars! They embraced the new healthy way of eating and lifestyle in a big way. Breeana dove right in—she learned to prepare healthy foods, began documenting everything, and the rest is history, as they say. I am excited to see her enthusiasm for this way of life paying off in ways other than her husband's now-resilient health.

Can I promise that if you embrace a lower refined sugar, low-allergen, anti-inflammatory diet rich in fruit and vegetables, in which the foods are mostly organic or sustainably raised, you will never get sick? No, but I do know that some of these measures are strongly supported by research and are known to help lower risks, especially for chronic disease like heart disease and diabetes. Lowering intake of pesticides as much as possible should also lower health risks for chronic diseases, when research clearly shows higher intakes increase risks for obesity and diabetes. Diet is just one part of a healthy lifestyle, but it certainly has a huge impact, right up there with not smoking and not sitting too much! Half the battle is figuring out how to stick with a healthier diet long-term. I have found the only way to do that is taking the time to prepare foods that are not only healthy, but that also taste great. In this way, we will want to eat them and can stick to a "healthy diet" as a long-term lifestyle. Breeana's recipes are stellar in that regard, and I can strongly recommend them as a great starting point for learning how to eat much healthier food.

Thank you, Breeana and Jason, for getting your story and message out there and encouraging and helping others to embrace and live healthier lives, starting with the quality of their food choices. It is my hope that as a result of you allowing me to write the foreword for this book, it will also help open the eyes of other health practitioners out there as to what truly can be accomplished in health-care with smart, well-researched nutritional support.

Yours in Health,
Jim LaValle

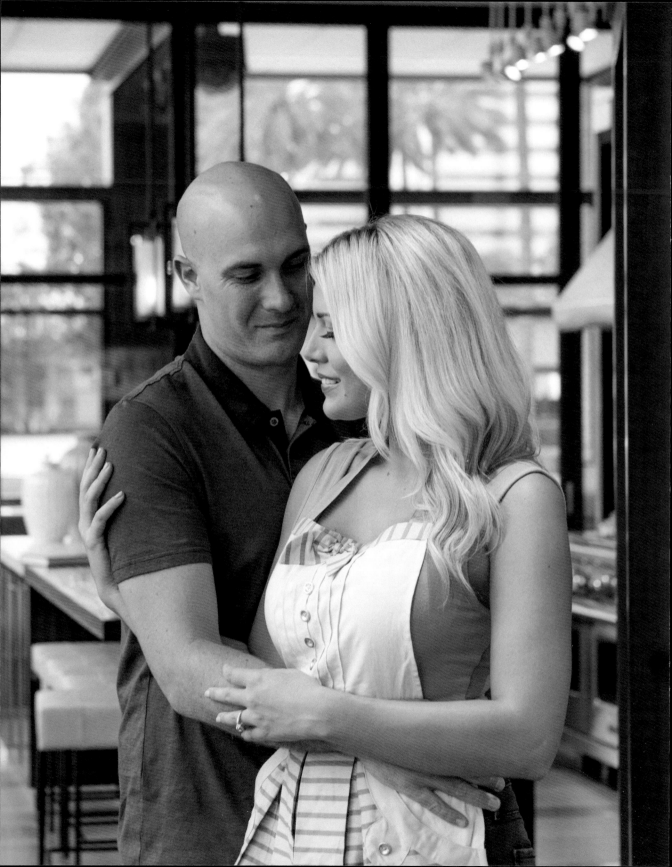

Introduction

I will never forget the day we found out my husband, Jason, had heart failure at the age of twenty-six. It is a memory so ingrained in my head, like a scene out of a movie. It felt like someone else's reality—not mine. How could this have happened to my healthy, active, twenty-six-year-old husband?

About four weeks prior to Jason's diagnosis of heart failure, his only symptom was this nagging cough he just couldn't get rid of. One day he came home from the gym and said it felt like someone had punched him in the chest, and the next day he had trouble breathing while playing basketball (something he did every week). So, we decided it was time he go and see a doctor.

We first went to a local urgent care where they diagnosed him with bronchitis, did a breathing treatment, and prescribed him an inhaler along with antibiotics. The urgent care told us it was nothing to be concerned about. After a week or so went by, Jason felt even worse after taking the antibiotics so I immediately made him an appointment to see his primary care doctor. The doctor examined him, noticed his elevated heart rate and very low blood pressure, and still told us he was fine and that some over-the-counter Robitussin should "do the trick."

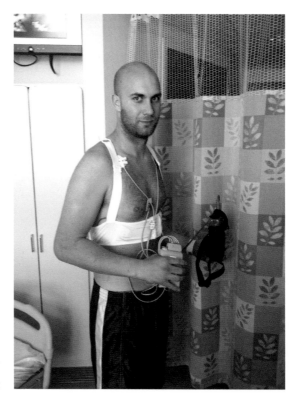

Another week went by and Jason's symptoms had not gotten any better, in fact his symptoms of coughing, chest pain, and difficulty breathing had only worsened—which is when I really started to worry.

We woke up on a Monday morning and Jason had no appetite and was feeling very weak, so I decided to take him to urgent care once more. They took his vitals and it again showed elevated heart rate and very low blood pressure. The urgent care doctor told us not to worry, that she thought his bronchitis had simply turned into a mild case of pneumonia. She told us she would prescribe a new dose of antibiotics, another inhaler, and a second breathing treatment. At that point I knew something was wrong, so I insisted on Jason at least getting a chest x-ray to make sure his heart and lungs were okay. The doctor said she did not think a chest x-ray was necessary, but she would do one "just for our peace of mind."

Within fifteen minutes of leaving the urgent care, the doctor called us with the chest x-ray results and said the x-ray showed that Jason's heart was very enlarged (cardiomyopathy) and that he needed to make an appointment to see his primary care doctor right away. With so much confusion and having no idea what cardiomyopathy even was,

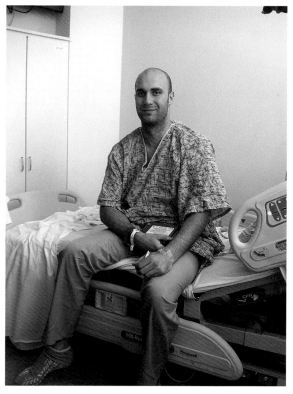

we drove directly to Jason's primary care doctor's office in a panic. His primary care doctor was faxed the chest x-ray results and after his doctor read the results he ordered an EKG to check Jason's heart. I still remember looking at that EKG machine and watching the results print out of it with bold letters at the top reading ABNORMAL. My stomach sank.

His doctor looked at the EKG results and said, "looks fine to me," then began to tell us the chest x-ray was not accurate because it must have been taken at a bad angle. He then prescribed Jason a heart medication to bring down his elevated heart rate, but told us other than that, we had nothing to worry about. Once again, we left the doctor's office with a feeling of hopelessness and utter confusion. All Jason's symptoms were pointing to something, yet his doctors kept telling us he was fine and prescribing him new medications to blanket over an obvious underlying issue.

The next morning, Jason's color was off. He looked almost gray, with this yellowish hue, and he still had no appetite which was not like him. I knew he needed some sort of nutrition—I made him a chicken noodle soup and almost instantly after eating it, he leaned over the kitchen sink and began to throw it up. I was standing in the living room watching him and when he turned around, he had to grab hold of the island in the center of our kitchen so he didn't fall over and faint. I knew in my gut something was terribly wrong, and I needed to take him to the emergency room. At first Jason refused, but after some convincing I finally got him in the car and drove off to the emergency room, not knowing what road lay ahead of us.

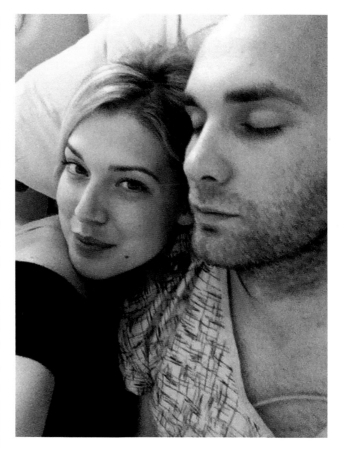

Within thirty minutes of being in the emergency room they ran blood work, did another EKG, and then performed an echocardiogram, which is an ultrasound of the heart. I'll never forget the look on Jason's face as he was lying in the hospital bed, dressed in that oversized hospital gown and his face so pale and grey. As we were anxiously waiting for his test results, I told him I would be back in a minute. As I walked to the restroom, the doctor who had been treating him saw me and gently grabbed my arm and said, "I don't know how to tell you this, but your husband has congestive heart failure. We are admitting him to the hospital immediately and need to find out what's going on with his heart and how this could have happened." I was in complete shock. What did that even mean? Congestive heart failure? How could this be possible?

I stayed in the hospital that night with Jason. They had a foldout chair that turned into a small bed and the nurse brought me some blankets. I don't think I slept one minute that night. My mind was racing and spinning, and we were still so confused on what his diagnosis actually meant.

Finally, the next morning the cardiologist came in to consult with Jason. The first thing the cardiologist said when he walked in the room was, "I don't know what the emergency room doctor told you guys, but I'm not going to sugarcoat anything. Jason, you have severe cardiomyopathy. Your echocardiogram shows you have an ejection fraction (the percentage at which your heart functions at) of about 9–10 percent. A normal ejection fraction is anywhere between 55–75 percent. Our goal is to find out what is causing the cardiomyopathy and make sure you don't have any blood clots or some type of blockage in your heart." After he spoke, the room was dead silent. We were at a complete loss for words.

The cardiologist believed his heart condition could have been viral, but since there was no way to prove this, his diagnosis became idiopathic cardiomyopathy, or heart failure caused from an unknown origin. He told us that what happened to Jason was so rare that it was a one in a million chance. He said not to worry about what had caused the cardiomyopathy because the damage was already done and what we needed to focus on was repairing his heart and bringing up the numbers on his ejection fraction.

He placed an external defibrillator on Jason that he had to wear at all times, except when showering, and this would monitor his heart in case he were to suddenly have a heart attack. The defibrillator would shock him, sending electro-waves into his chest if he happened to go into cardiac arrest.

Once they fit Jason for his defibrillator, I remember walking out of his hospital room only to see the waiting room filled with about thirty of our closest family and friends. My eyes filled with tears, and I began sobbing just thinking of everything we had learned the past few days, and being so unsure of Jason's future.

After being in the hospital about a week, Jason was discharged and released with various heart medications and the defibrillator. Before leaving, his cardiologist told us Jason was at risk of having a heart attack and dying at any moment because of his extremely low ejection fraction. He told us he had no idea if Jason's heart would repair itself, that only time could tell, and if Jason's ejection fraction was not up to 35 percent in three months' time he would need a pacemaker surgically inserted and would also be put on a heart transplant list. The words "heart transplant" really

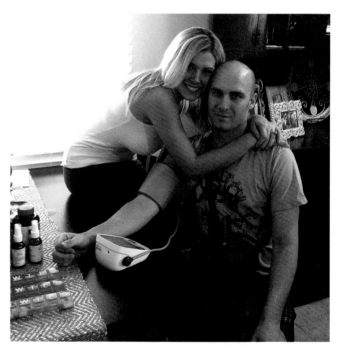

struck a chord with us. It felt so surreal, like an out-of-body experience. Upon leaving the hospital, the cardiologist gave us little to no hope for Jason's future and told us to "play things by ear." He sent us off with a stack of prescriptions and told us his only diet restrictions were to reduce his sodium intake.

Day in and day out, Jason rested at home with no signs of improvement. I remember lying on his chest at night before we went to bed to listen to his heart beat. His heart was beating so fast it sounded like it was going to jump out of his chest. Every night, I was so afraid of waking up the next morning and Jason not being alive.

My mother suggested that Jason meet with a naturopath clinician one of her friends had recommended. Jason was extremely reluctant at first, but knew he needed to try anything to save his life. We consulted with the naturopath clinician James LaValle. After hearing of Jason's symptoms and diagnosis, he told us Jason needed to be on an anti-inflammatory diet to help bring down the inflammation in his heart. The anti-inflammatory diet consisted of gluten-free, dairy-free, and all organic foods. He told us it was imperative for Jason to go organic to help rid his body of excess toxins and preservatives and that gluten and dairy both cause inflammation in the body, which we needed to keep down as much as possible. He also said Jason needed to eat a lot of organic animal protein, as the heart is a muscle and the quickest way to build muscle is through protein. He also specified to avoid processed food and refined sugar—so basically no junk food or fast food, just a completely clean, organic diet. He put Jason on a strict vitamin and supplement plan with what he felt his body needed to heal and in turn help speed up the healing process. He had Jason take a test that sent electrodes through his system by testing different pressure points on his body, and those pressure points told him what vitamins Jason's system reacted well to. We also found out through this process that Jason was in fact severely allergic to gluten.

Dr. LaValle told us he knew Jason could beat this and he was going to make sure my husband didn't need that heart transplant. I left his office that day, feeling for the first time a kernel of hope in this war to try and save my husband's life in such a short amount of time.

Let me start out by saying Jason is the pickiest eater on the planet, so this new diet came with a load of challenges and obstacles, but we were willing to try anything. After our appointment with James, I threw out everything in our refrigerator and pantry, went grocery shopping, and decided to give this one hundred percent of my time, energy, and passion.

I've always enjoyed cooking. I would never consider myself a Master Chef, but I've always considered myself an avid foodie who enjoys a great meal. After Jason and I were married in 2010, I started watching the Food Network, reading cookbooks, and picking

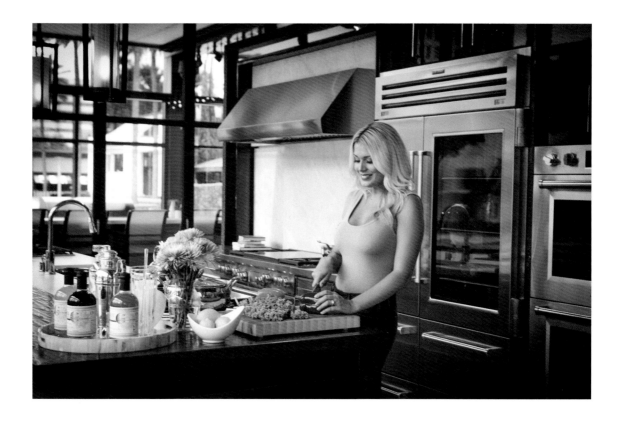

up tips wherever I could. Slowly but surely, my cooking skills improved and it became something I found therapy in. My real passion for cooking, however, came after Jason's diagnosis, and I learned the true meaning of how food can heal the body.

I started to create recipes to help heal Jason's heart. I wanted to find a way to make this healthy food I was feeding him not taste so bland. I decided document our journey and share my recipes with others who might be struggling with their own health issues, or for people who just needed some healthy recipe ideas.

Gradually, I started to see a huge change in Jason's health and appearance. At first, it was his color that came back. He wasn't that grey and yellowish color I had become so accustomed to. Then he started to move around more, he felt like going on walks, and he wasn't as tired all the time. It was so amazing to be able to see the little changes in his progress every day.

I started to realize that I could turn what some might consider a tragedy into something truly positive. Since Jason was on disability and not really able to leave the house, or drive a car for that matter, I put all my energy into taking care of him and making his illness as fun as possible (sounds strange, I know). Jason was sick, yes, but he at least was getting fed amazing, home-cooked meals that brightened his day, and in turn, cooking became the most exciting part of my day. I really started to experiment with food, and what came out of that was amazing. I felt like for the first time I found myself, my calling—the only thing I've ever been this passionate about in my entire life.

Creating healthy meals that are full of nutrients to heal your body, but that also taste like delicious, gourmet, savory foods. And what's funny is, I actually became pretty good at this cooking thing!

Every day, I experimented with new recipes. I entered the exciting world of gluten-free and all the obstacles that came along with it. Who knew that gluten is in just about everything in the entire world? So that meant experimenting with new, foreign ingredients, and really doing my homework on how I can make this plain food actually taste good. I really began to enjoy the challenge of experimenting with new flavors.

Before we knew it, Jason's dreaded three-month checkup had arrived with his cardiologist, the one who had previously told us if his heart's ejection fraction was not at 35 percent in three months' time he would need a heart transplant. We were so nervous going into this appointment, I don't think we ever let go of each other's hands the whole time. We really had no idea what to expect. All we knew was Jason was feeling better each day, and we prayed that his test result numbers would show just that. After they performed the echocardiogram, we anxiously waited in the doctor's office for the test results. The cardiologist finally walked in and told us his ejection fraction was at 35 percent. You can imagine how thrilled we were, we both burst into tears. His cardiologist told us that Jason was a miracle, and he in no way expected these types of numbers in such a short amount of time.

Every few months, Jason would get a new echocardiogram and his numbers just kept rising. Every day he felt better, had more energy, and began to feel like himself again. We stuck with the eating plan James LaValle had recommended to us from the beginning, and that eating plan turned into a way of life for us.

Flash forward two-and-a-half years and Jason no longer needs a heart transplant—better yet, he is healthier than he has ever been in his entire life and his heart is now within normal range. Jason went from not being able to walk halfway through Target because he was so weak and tired, to now being able to run and play basketball every day. His doctors, who had given us little hope for the future, began calling him a modern-day miracle, but we knew it was not a miracle. Food truly saved Jason's life.

I decided to make it my mission to share our story and my recipes that healed Jason with others, and I knew creating this cookbook would help spread my message. This was no easy task, and I knew it was going to take a lot of determination for me to get a cookbook published. After getting turned down by dozens of literary agents, I finally got signed with an agency who believed in my work and the message I was spreading. That agency quickly found a publisher who wanted to publish my cookbook and make my dream a reality.

I hope all of you enjoy this cookbook as much as I've enjoyed making it. This cookbook is my heart, and not one second of making it ever felt like work to me, but instead it felt like I was finally doing what I was always meant to do.

—Breeana

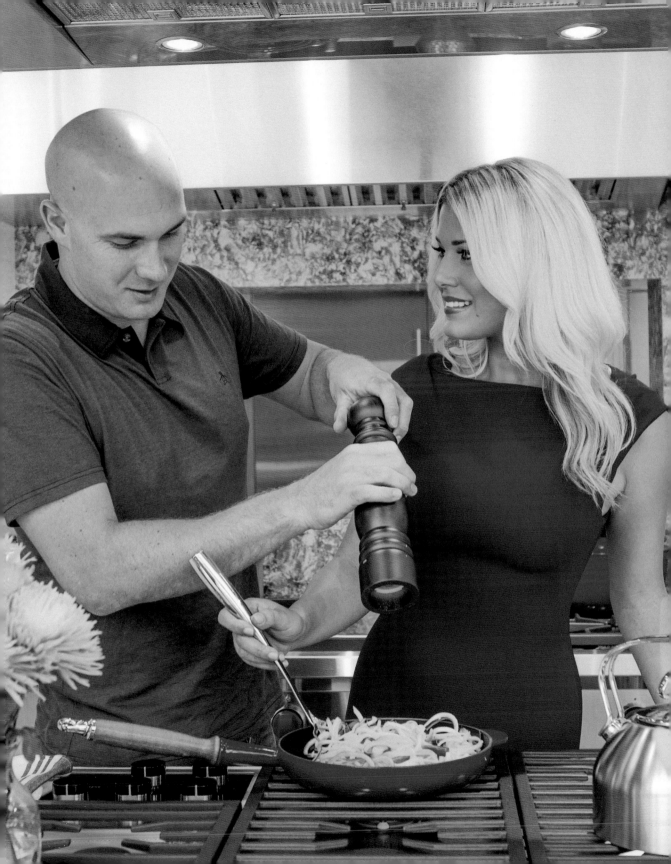

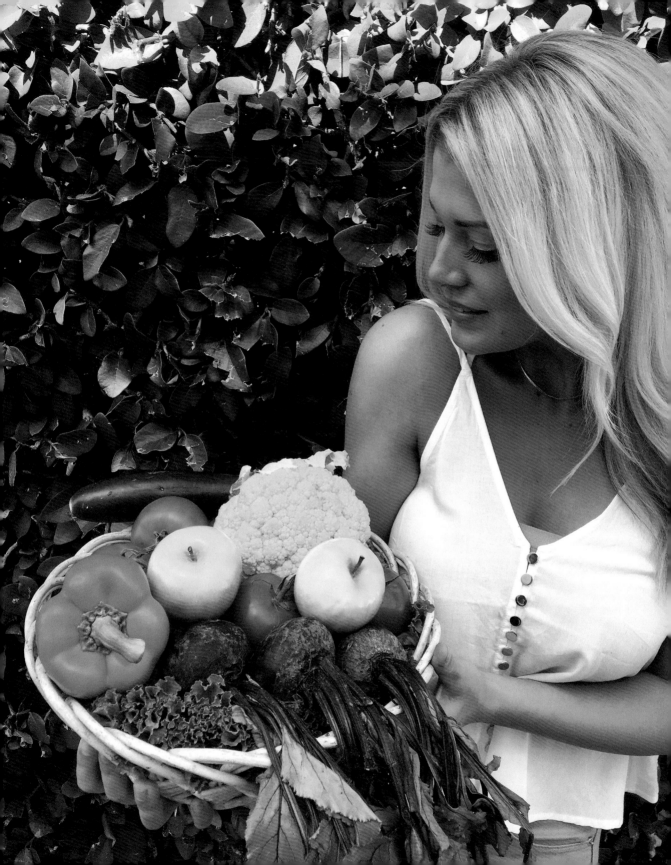

Changing Health Through Food

Food Revolution—Count Chemicals, Not Calories

I remember the days in my not-so-distant past where I thought eating a Special-K Protein Bar or a Slim Fast Shake as a meal replacement made me healthy. Sure, they may be low in calories, have some sort of protein on the nutrition label, and be advertised on television as a healthy meal replacement, but what really is healthy? What truly makes a person healthy?

I think one of the biggest misconceptions of our generation is what type of food is actually good for us. Ten years ago, most people didn't think about chemicals in their food. They didn't think to check the ingredients label, but instead society had taught us to only look at the nutrition label—how many calories are in each serving of this cereal? How many grams of carbs? And oh *dear*, look at the fat content! What we didn't realize was, maybe we didn't even need to be looking at the nutrition label. Why? When you eat real food, food that is free of chemicals and additives, free of harmful preservatives, of food coloring and dyes, food that isn't made from the same chemical that your yoga mat in the garage is made from (a.k.a. azodicarbonamide, a substance commonly used at fast-food restaurants that conditions dough to make it more elastic), you don't need to look at the nutrition label.

When you nourish your body with real food (like a whole organic potato purchased at the grocery store, instead of McDonalds fries which contain twelve ingredients), you no longer need to worry about calories. By eating real food, you are supplying your body with actual nutrients. Nutrients derived from their original source, not depleted nutrients created in a lab. Real food contains nutrients that your body is able to fully process and benefit from the enriched vitamins and protein that it so desperately needs to function.

So here's a thought—why not try and completely remove these processed foods from our lives so our bodies can function at their maximum capacity? Seems simple, right? *Wrong*. Not when you live in a society where most corporate companies are trying to cut costs at every corner, and incorporating these chemicals and additives into our food makes producing their products not only cheaper, but they also make the product last longer. So what is one to do in a world filled with processed foods that are taunting us at every corner?

Try this:

1. Buy as much organic food as possible. While it's not always possible to eat organic 100 percent of the time, when you do eat organic it vastly eliminates the toxins and pesticides in your body.
2. Focus on only reading the ingredients label and paying more attention to what actually goes into your food. The less ingredients listed, the better (unless of course the ingredients are mostly seasonings, etc.).
3. Go out to eat as little as possible and cook at home more. Obviously, we want to live a balanced life, and there is nothing wrong with going out to eat and splurging, but save this for special occasions. And for those who say they are too busy to cook at home, you can meal prep on Sundays for the whole week! They even have organic meal prep companies that will do this for you and drop the food off at your doorstep. It doesn't get much more simple than that.

Genetically Modified Organisms, a.k.a. GMOs

GMOs are something I didn't even know existed before Jason's diagnosis. Let's clarify, because there is a lot of confusion around the topic.

Genetically Modified Organism: when a gene from one organism is purposely moved to improve or change another organism in a lab, the result is a GMO. So in layman's terms, the DNA of our food is changed in a lab to make our food "better"—better how? It optimizes agricultural performance and makes it easier for farmers to grow, increases crop yields, reduces production costs, reduces needs for pesticides (because the pesticides are already built into the crop seed), and can actually enhance the food quality and make it taste better.

Example: Have you ever bought an organic apple at the grocery store? They tend to be small and have bruises all over. Now compare it to an apple that is derived from a GMO crop seed—that apple is bigger, nice and shiny, and you can't find one bruise on the thing. Get the picture?

So, if GMOs make it so much easier for farmers, then why are they not good for us? Consider this—most developed nations do not consider GMOs to be safe. In fact, in more than sixty countries around the world, GMOs are actually banned. In the United States, the only GMO-based studies that have been conducted are in fact done by the same companies that created GMOs and benefit from their multi-billion dollar sales.

GMOs have been studied in other countries, and they've caused rats to develop horrifying tumors, organ damage, and premature death. Some scientists and researchers believe GMOs are linked to many forms of cancer and disease in humans,

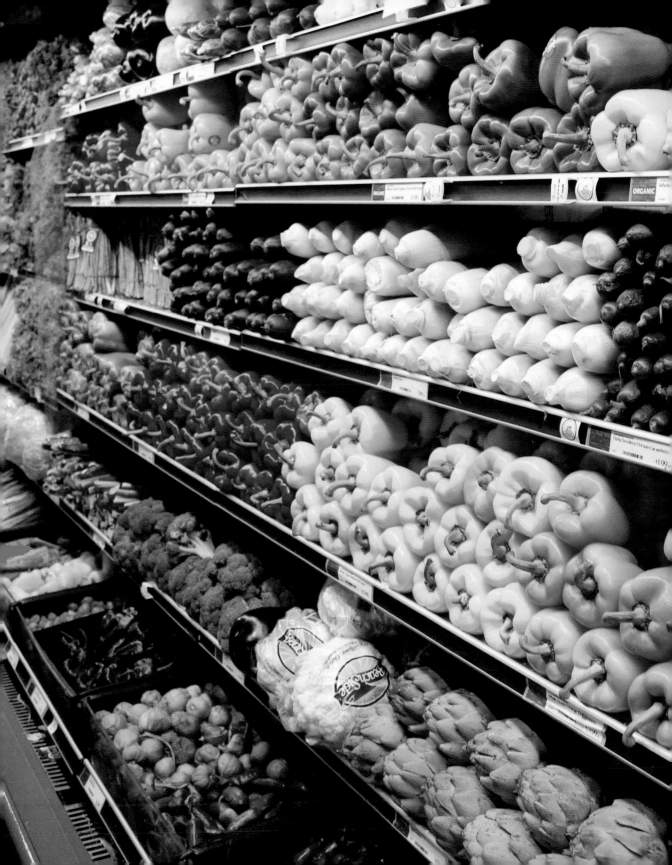

too. Would you rather have your food's DNA designed by humans and artificially changed in a lab, or have food that was grown in the ground the good old-fashioned way, as humans have been doing for thousands of years?

The wonderful part about eating organic foods is they can never contain GMOs, according to FDA regulation. So, if you buy organic foods you don't ever have to worry about GMOs and how potentially harmful they could be to your body. Bottom line—when in doubt if something contains GMOs, just go the organic route.

How to Go Organic and Not Break the Bank

The most common thing I hear from people is purchasing organic food is too expensive and they just can't afford it. And trust me, when we first learned of Jason's diagnosis and we were told he needed to eat a completely organic diet, our grocery bills doubled. That's right, *doubled.*

What I came to realize is that if going organic is truly important to us and something that I know could potentially save my husband's life (plus, is way better for our health long-term), then how is money even in the equation? What I had to do was make other little sacrifices in our lives so that we could afford this newly organic lifestyle. This meant not always buying that new pair of shoes, skipping out on that concert I really wanted to go to, and going out to eat less often. I previously discussed how important it is to cook at home, and what's amazing is when you cook at home more and go out to eat less, you'll notice your food bills will equal out to about the same. So ask yourself, can you really put a price on your health? If you don't have your health, let's face it, you don't have anything. So, make those little sacrifices so you can afford to buy mostly organic food.

Now you may ask, is eating organic actually better for your health? Studies show that by switching to an organic food lifestyle, it will rapidly eliminate pesticide residue in your body and in turn you will begin to rid your body of all those unwanted stored toxins and free radicals (toxic byproducts of oxygen that can cause significant damage to living cells).

I've always said that people who don't believe in the organic eating trend of our generation are people who have not yet educated themselves on food today. Nutrient density has declined approximately 40–60 percent over the past hundred years and continues to decline. That means our food today typically has 50 percent fewer nutrients than the same food had a hundred years ago. Studies show that organically grown foods generate more nutrients and fewer nitrates. In a study comparing organic and conventionally grown food (done by the Soil Association Certification Ltd.), they reported that organic crops were much higher in essential minerals, phytonutrients (enzymes, antioxidants, and bioflavonoids), and vitamin C. Meaning, organic food does actually have more nutrients—nutrients your body could be benefiting from and that your body could be using to heal itself.

Here are a few simple tips I've found that can help cut costs when purchasing organic foods:

1. Comparison shop—By shopping around at different grocery stores you'll get a general idea for which organic foods are less costly at certain stores, or which location offers the most deals overall.
2. Create your weekly meal plans based around what organic produce/meats/grains are on sale that week.
3. Improvise—If an organic ingredient isn't available or affordable you might find something else that works just as well, or even better, than the original ingredient.
4. Invest in bulk organic meats and produce—Buy your items in bulk and freeze for later use. Buying organic products in bulk can greatly decrease costs.
5. Support your local organic farmers—Buy directly from your local farmers to save money. Most cities have weekly farmer's markets where local farmers offer great organic items, typically at a lower cost. You can even bargain with them! Two for one?
6. Select seasonal produce—Buy whatever organic produce item is in season and plan your meals around that. Seasonal produce is typically much cheaper since it's more readily available at that time.

By choosing to live a mostly organic lifestyle, you'll notice the results almost immediately in how much better you feel. We, unfortunately, live in a day and age where our foods are so processed and filled with chemicals that eating organic is imperative.

I once had someone tell me that they think eating organic is completely ridiculous and their grandparents lived well into their nineties and never ate organic and were "just fine." I just laughed, because what they didn't realize is the food their grandparents ate fifty, sixty, years ago is not the same as the food we eat today. Not only are the nutrients in food more depleted today, but GMOs didn't exist, food wasn't as processed, and they didn't use the chemicals present in food now.

I can't even begin to stress the importance of educating yourself on this topic. There are so many books, documentaries, and websites that contain countless hours of research on the powerful healing methods of food and the importance of going organic. So use your resources, educate yourself on the

See my resource list on page 184 to help you get started!

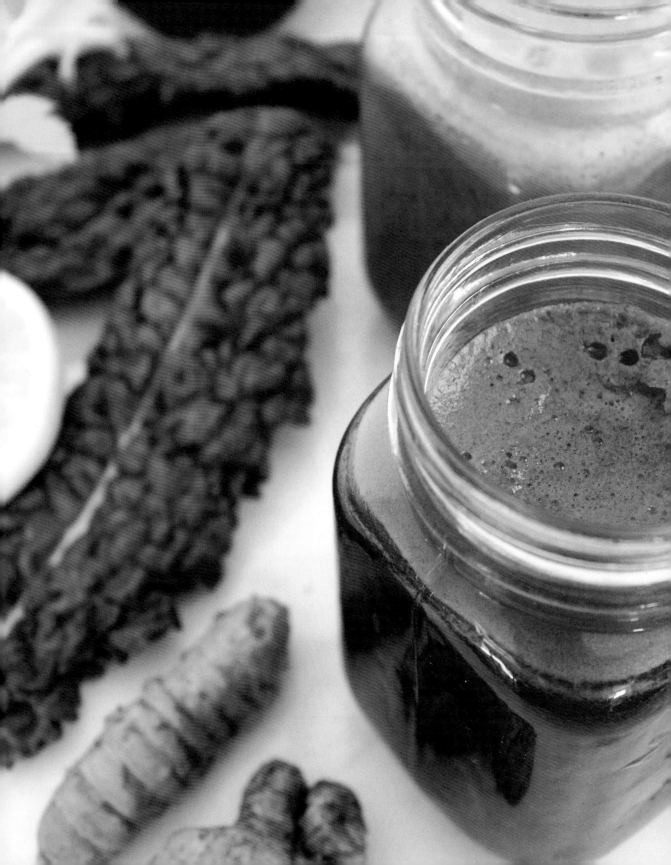

topic, and come to your own conclusion on the matter. I guarantee once you do this, you'll never want to buy conventional food products again!

Using Food as Medicine

One thing I would like to point out is this book is in no way, shape, or form, a book about dieting, how to lose weight, or counting your macros—it's actually opposite of that. This book is the story of how my husband overcame heart failure and the recipes I made to help heal him in the process. What happened to Jason was such an eye-opener for us both and made us take a magnifying glass to our food choices and how we chose to live our lives. It caused us to do so much research on the topics of food, and of health, and of organic and unprocessed foods. I actually saw before my own eyes my husband fighting for his life, and within a week of changing his food habits, his symptoms started to improve.

By using food as medicine, you are providing your body with a surplus of nutrients that are packed full of vitamins and antioxidants that your body needs to function at its highest peak. Our bodies are designed to heal themselves. That's why when you fall and scrape your knee, your body instantly starts creating a scab to cover over the wound, to protect it and heal from the inside out. So why would any other injury or disease be different?

Studies show that inflammation in your body is where disease thrives and breeds. By bringing down the inflammation in your system, your body can focus on healing itself. When your body is inflamed, it's almost like you're at war with yourself. Your body is constantly trying to fight off pesticides and toxins that are stored in your system through chemicals and processed foods. When you vastly eliminate these harmful substances from your body and eat foods that fight inflammation, your body is able to focus on healing, instead of fighting itself.

If you take anything away from this cookbook, I want you to take away these four simple points:

1. Focus on buying foods at their closest natural source.
2. Eat organic as much as possible.
3. Count chemicals, not calories.
4. Always do your own research and educate yourself, no matter what anyone tells you.

Always remember—you don't need to be a spectacular cook to create healthy and delicious meals. Practice, practice, practice, and you'll be amazed at how fast you catch on and in turn, how therapeutic it can become for you, just as it was for me.

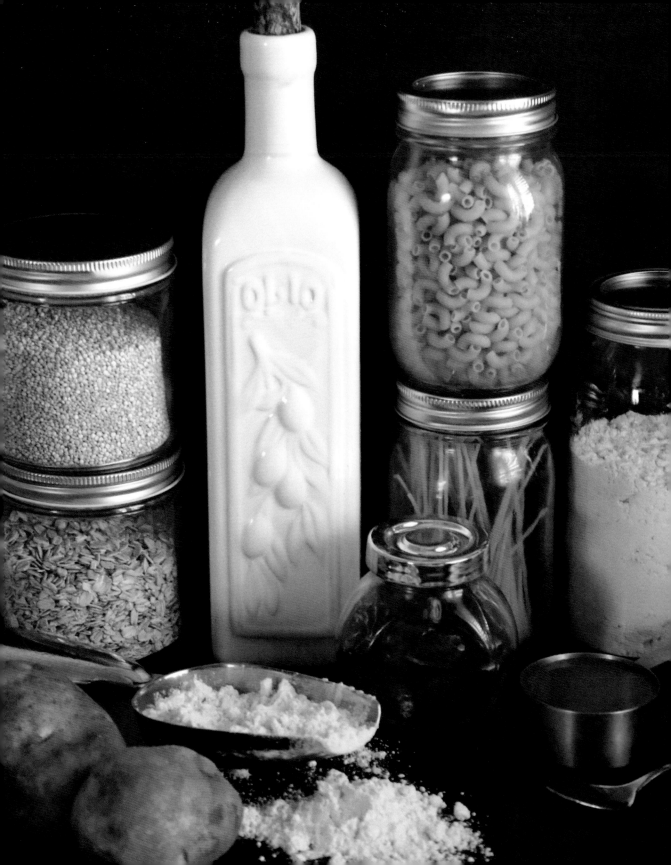

The Gluten- and Dairy-Free Kitchen and Pantry

Here is a list of everything you will need for the recipes in this book. You'll find I use a lot of seasonings in my recipes. You don't have to be an amazing cook, but if you learn the art of seasoning, it will take your food to a whole new level. If one of my recipes looks long and difficult, you'll find that most of the ingredients listed are seasonings and are part of the average home pantry! Not to say I don't use a few ingredients that aren't as common, such as coconut aminos or tahini, but even these ingredients can be found at your local grocery store.

As mentioned in the beginning chapters, always try to opt for the organic option if it's available and read your ingredients labels when shopping for groceries. The goal is to eat your food as unprocessed and as close to its original source as possible with minimal additives and preservatives.

So, I've created this shopping list for you to get started on your journey to the world of gluten- and dairy-free cooking.

Dried Herbs, Spices, and Seasonings:

These are my ride-or-die seasonings that I always keep stocked in my pantry.

- Garlic powder
- Onion powder
- Cinnamon
- Nutmeg
- Paprika
- Cumin
- Chili powder
- Curry powder
- Ground mustard
- Coarse salt (such as sea salt)
- Coarse black pepper
- Crushed red pepper
- Cayenne pepper
- Coriander
- White peppercorn
- Bay leaves

Herbs I Always Use Fresh:

So far, the only herb I've successfully grown is rosemary (and just about anyone can grow that). As Jason would say, I was not blessed with a green thumb! It's great if you can grow a fresh herb garden at home, but if not, you can buy organic herbs at any grocery store at a minimal cost.

- Italian flat leaf parsley
- Basil
- Cilantro
- Thyme
- Rosemary
- Chives
- Mint
- Sage

Canned and Pantry Goods:

When it comes to items like broths and tomato sauces, always go for the low-sodium option. You want to be able to control how much or how little sodium you add to a dish.

- Chicken, beef, or vegetable broth
- Crushed tomatoes, tomato sauce, tomato paste
- Raw peanut and almond butter
- Tahini paste
- Raw almonds, cashews, walnuts
- Sesame seeds, pumpkin seeds, flax seeds, chia seeds
- Coconut shreds (unsweetened)
- Almond meal
- Green chili peppers
- Water chestnuts
- Active dry yeast packets, nutritional yeast flakes
- Baking soda
- Protein powder

Dairy-Free Milk Alternatives:

My go-to milk alternatives are usually almond or coconut milk. I am not a fan of soy milk (even if it is organic). Soy is highly processed and has a funky aftertaste which doesn't translate well when cooking with it. I always try to make my almond milk homemade, as most store-bought almond milks contain a lot of additives and preservatives. I also prefer to buy my coconut milk in a can. Most coconut milk in a can contains guar gum, which is fine since it's all-natural. Guar gum comes from a seed that is ground and milled and used as a thickening agent in foods.

- Full-fat and light coconut milk
- Almond milk (recipe on page 115)

Gluten-Free Grains, Flours, and Pastas:

It's so simple nowadays to find gluten-free pastas and flours at any grocery store. Luckily, rice and quinoa are naturally gluten-free. Even though something is labeled gluten-free, it's still important to check the ingredients label. Gluten-free products can sneak in harmful chemicals and artificial flavors.

- Brown rice, Arborio rice
- Quinoa
- Gluten-free noodles: fettucine, elbow macaroni, lasagna sheets, pad-Thai or rice noodles
- Gluten-free gnocchi
- Corn tortillas (check your ingredients as some may still contain wheat)
- Rolled oats
- All-purpose gluten-free flour:
  - Bob's Red Mill gluten-free all-purpose flour (you can find this brand at most grocery stores)
  - Bob's Red Mill gluten-free one-on-one flour
  - gluten-free organic flour blend (this brand is available in some stores, but if you can't find it in a store just purchase it online. It's the absolute best gluten-free flour for baking)
- Rice paper wraps
- Rice crackers
- Cornmeal (always buy organic cornmeal to avoid GMOs)
- Gluten-free panko bread crumbs
- Gluten-free pre-made pizza crusts

Meats, Poultry, and Fish:

If you are going to buy anything organic, always try and buy your meats, poultry, and fish organic and wild-caught. Especially when it comes to bacon, make sure it's all-natural, uncured, and preferably sugar-free. If you don't eat red meat, you can substitute any ground beef recipe for ground turkey or chicken. If you don't eat meat or any kind of animal by-products, you will find it simple to make any of my recipes vegan or vegetarian-friendly by removing just a few simple ingredients.

- Ground beef, steaks such as rib eye or New York strips
- Chicken breasts, chicken wings, chicken sausage, rotisserie chicken (Whole Foods sells organic rotisserie chicken that is perfect for quick meals)
- Eggs
- Ground turkey, deli-style turkey meat
- Salmon, halibut, and shrimp
- Bacon

Fruits, Vegetables, Plants, and Legumes:

If you can't afford to buy all of your produce organic, my rule of thumb is to always buy produce organic if it has flesh you're biting directing into. For instance, lettuce, raspberries, and apples I always buy organic. Items such as bananas, avocados, and spaghetti squash aren't as high on the priority list because you do not eat the skin, therefore the flesh is not as compromised with pesticides' chemicals.

- Raspberries
- Frozen pitaya smoothie packs
- Bananas
- Pineapple
- Mangos
- Blueberries
- Unsweetened raisins
- Pink lady apples, green apples
- Oranges
- Roma, heirloom, and cherry tomatoes
- Avocados
- Lemons, limes
- Tomatillos
- Cucumbers
- Mushrooms
- Green cabbage, purple cabbage
- Cauliflower (riced and the whole head)
- Green leaf, iceberg, and romaine lettuce
- Watercress
- Radicchio
- Collard greens
- Asparagus
- Jalapeño peppers (green and red), habanero peppers, Thai chili peppers
- Bell peppers
- Kale
- Spinach
- Brussels sprouts
- Russet potatoes, sweet potatoes
- Spaghetti, acorn, and butternut squash
- Celery
- Carrots
- Zucchinis
- Beets
- Yellow onions, sweet onions, red onions, green onions, shallots
- Garlic
- Ginger root, turmeric root
- Lemongrass stalks
- Mung bean sprouts
- Garbanzo beans (chickpeas)
- Sweet garden peas, sugar snap peas
- Peanuts

Oils and Vinegars:

I mostly use olive oil and coconut oil in my recipes. Mainly because I like the ways these oils taste when used for cooking and they are both healthy fats to incorporate into your daily diet.

- Extra-virgin olive oil
- Avocado oil (great for cooking those high-temperature foods)
- Virgin-unrefined coconut oil
- Non-stick cooking spray
- Sesame seed oil
- Apple cider vinegar
- Balsamic vinegar

Sweeteners, Condiments, and Sauces:

I never use white sugar (refined sugar) in any of my recipes. Refined sugar has no nutritional value, is highly processed with chemicals, and is usually bleached. Instead, I opt for raw sweeteners such as honey, maple syrup, or dates. These un-refined sweeteners have actual nutrients your body can retain, are easier for our bodies to digest, and are much less processed. However, sugar is sugar, so I always still use un-refined sugars in moderation.

- Raw honey
- Pitted dates
- 100 percent pure maple syrup
- Unsweetened applesauce
- Coconut aminos
- Ketchup (I use the Mama Jess garden ketchup—it's naturally sweetened with beets and plums!)
- Barbeque sauce (try and opt for an organic barbeque sauce sweetened with honey rather than refined sugars)
- Worcestershire sauce
- Frank's Red Hot sauce
- Sriracha sauce (recipe on page 128)
- Fresh salsa, hot sauce, chili sauce
- Stone ground, Dijon, and yellow mustard

Tools and Gadgets in the Kitchen:

These are the kitchen tools I use most often. I simply cannot live without my Dutch oven and you'll see that a lot of my recipes use one. A food processor is wonderful for creating homemade sauces and dips, and a high-power blender is necessary for recipes such as my pitaya bowl.

- Food processor
- High-power blender
- Juicer
- Vegetable spiralizer
- Dutch oven
- Cooling rack
- Electric hand mixer
- Nut milk bag
- Cheesecloth
- Good knife set

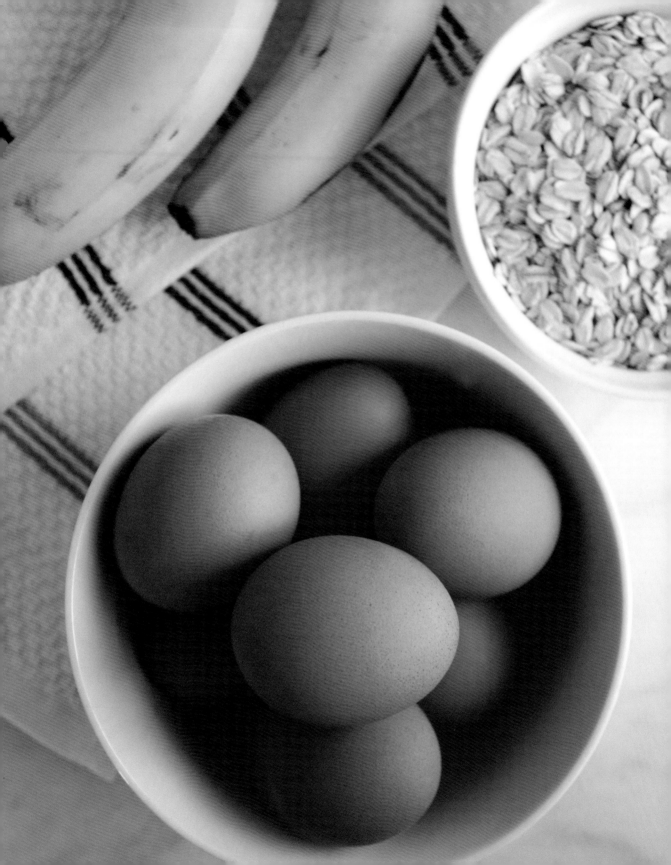

Breakfast

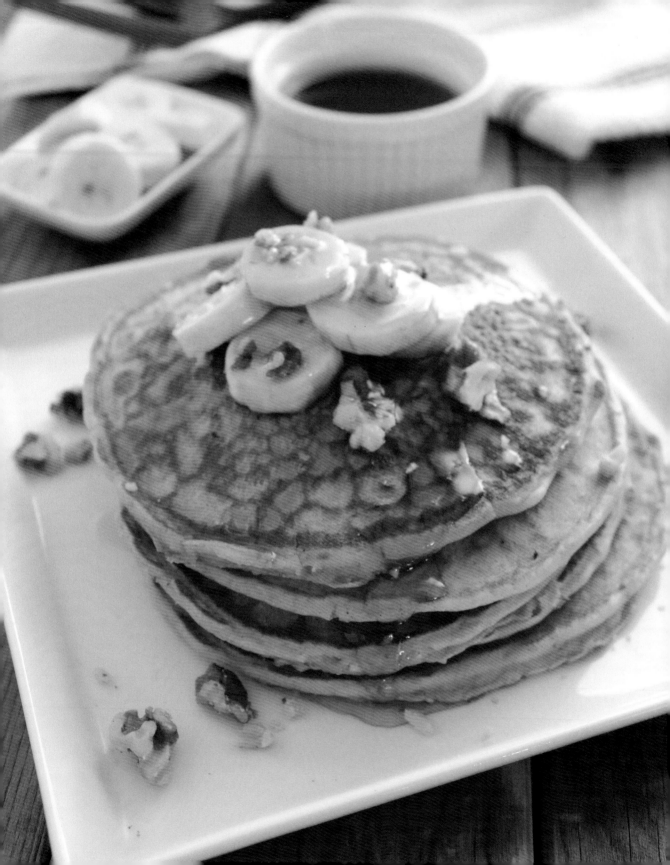

PANCAKES

Gluten-Free, Dairy-Free, Vegetarian

Makes 6–7 Pancakes

One of my favorite things to make on a cozy Sunday morning is pancakes. There is nothing more comforting than your family waking up to the smell of fresh, homemade pancakes. I've tried making gluten-free pancakes numerous times, every which way possible, and this is by far the best recipe. It's important to use full-fat coconut milk with this recipe because it really thickens the batter and gives the pancakes that fluffy texture. We like to top these with fresh bananas, walnuts, and pure maple syrup, but feel free to top them with whatever your heart desires!

1½ cups gluten-free all-purpose flour
½ teaspoon baking soda
½ teaspoon salt
¼ teaspoon cinnamon
1 teaspoon chia seeds
1½ cups full-fat coconut milk
2 eggs
1 tablespoon coconut oil
1 tablespoon honey

1. In a large bowl, mix together the dry ingredients. In a separate bowl, mix together the wet ingredients. Transfer the wet ingredients into dry ingredients and combine the batter well.

2. Grease a non-stick skillet with cooking spray and bring it to a medium heat. For each pancake, ladle the pancake batter onto the heated skillet and cook each side about 2 minutes.

3. Serve your pancakes topped with warmed, pure maple syrup or honey.

> **TIP:** I use the Bob's Red Mill 1-to-1 Gluten-Free Flour for the best pancake results.

SWEET POTATO TOAST

Gluten-Free, Dairy-Free, Grain-Free, Vegan

Makes 6 Toasts (2–3 Servings)

These decedent sweet potato toasts are incredible for breakfast—or anytime of the day, really. The crisp sweet potatoes topped with the luscious macadamia cream cheese and a sweet and tangy radicchio salad is the perfect combination.

1 large sweet potato
2 tablespoons coconut oil
⅓ cup macadamia cream cheese
*   (recipe on page 111)*
1½ avocados, sliced thin
¼ teaspoon salt
Black pepper, as desired
Pinch of crushed red pepper

Radicchio Salad:
1 tablespoon lemon juice
1 tablespoon maple syrup
1 teaspoon apple cider vinegar
1 cup roughly chopped watercress
1 cup shredded radicchio

1. Preheat your oven to 450 degrees. Line a baking sheet with aluminum foil, then place a cooling rack over the baking sheet.

2. Slice the ends off the sweet potato then cut it lengthwise into 6 equal ¼-inch pieces. It's important to make sure the pieces are all cut as evenly as possible so they cook at the same time. Brush each side of the sweet potatoes in coconut oil. Place the sweet potatoes on the cooling rack and bake for 10 minutes, then flip them over and bake an additional 5–10 minutes or until the edges are crispy and the sweet potato is cooked through. Remove the sweet potato slices from the oven.

3. In a small bowl, mix together the lemon juice, maple syrup, and apple cider vinegar. Toss the watercress and radicchio in the dressing.

4. Spread the macadamia cream cheese equally on each toast then top with the avocado slices and sprinkle the tops with salt, pepper, and crushed red pepper. Top with the salad.

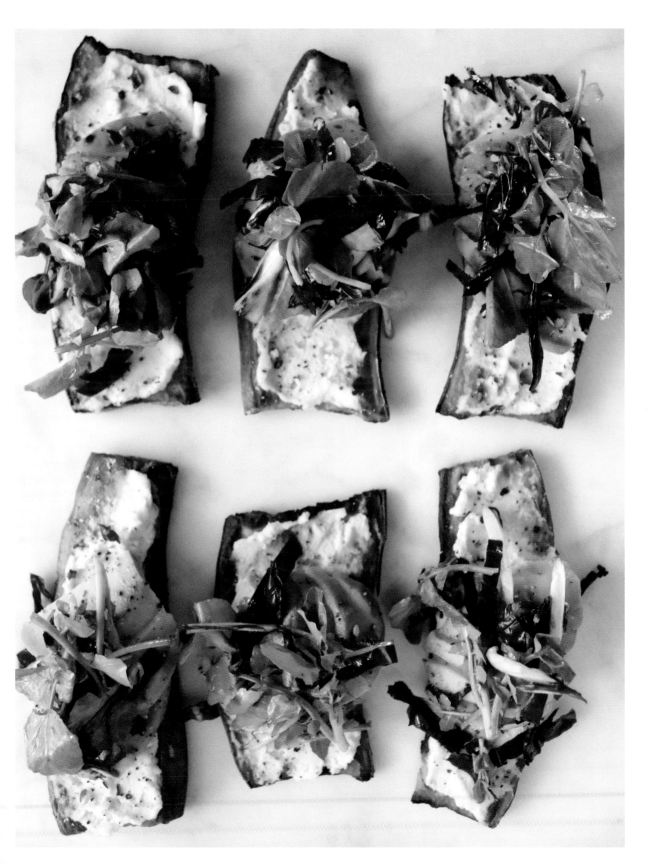

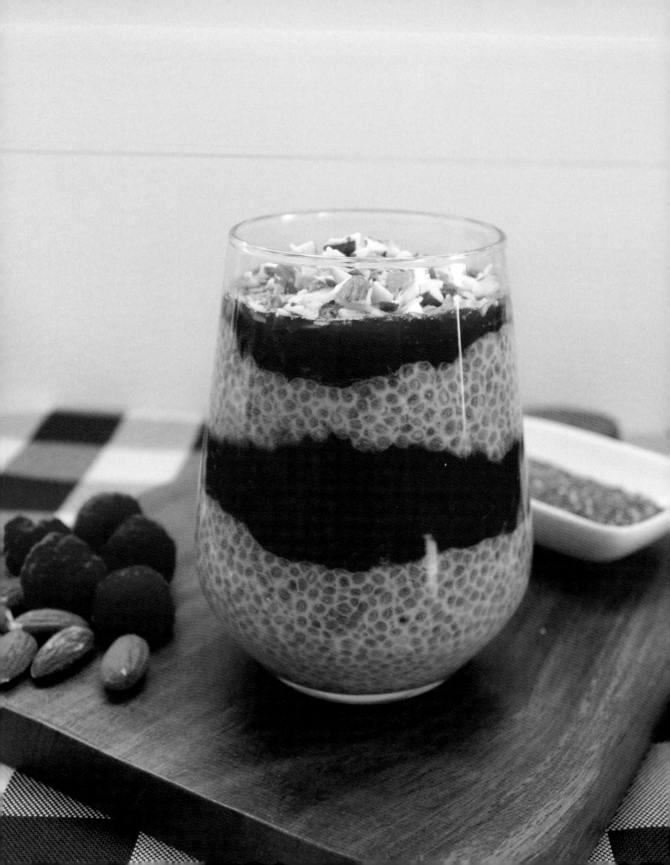

RASPBERRY-ALMOND CHIA SEED PARFAIT

Gluten-Free, Dairy-Free, Grain-Free, Vegetarian

1–2 Servings

I love this for breakfast because you can prepare the chia seed pudding the night before and the raspberry sauce takes less than a minute to make. If you haven't tried chia seed pudding I highly recommend making this! The chia seeds become gelatinous and expand which is what turns it into a pudding-like texture. And the simple raspberry sauce is the icing on the cake.

Chia Seed Pudding:
3 tablespoons chia seeds
1 cup unsweetened almond milk
1½ tablespoons honey
¼ teaspoon cinnamon

Raspberry Sauce:
1 cup fresh raspberries
½ tablespoon honey
Zest from ½ small lemon

Toppings:
1–2 tablespoons crushed almonds
Unsweetened coconut shreds, as desired

1. In a bowl mix together the chia seeds, almond milk, honey, and cinnamon, making sure everything is well combined. Cover the bowl and let it sit in the refrigerator overnight.

2. For the raspberry sauce, in a food processor puree the fresh raspberries, honey, and lemon zest until completely smooth.

3. To assemble the parfait in a mason jar or glass, layer the chia seed pudding with the raspberry sauce. Top the parfait with crushed almonds and coconut shreds.

> **FACT:** Chia seeds are packed full of fiber, protein, and antioxidants. Chia seeds expand in your stomach and actually make you feel full longer!

KALE AND BACON FRITTATA WITH CRISPY SHALLOTS

Gluten-Free, Dairy-Free, Grain-Free

4–5 Servings

This frittata is wonderful to serve at a brunch with friends or to eat throughout the week. Jason is such a picky eater when it comes to vegetables, but for some reason he adores kale so this recipe has become a go-to for us in the mornings. And let me tell you, the crispy shallots that top the frittata are *everything*. This casserole is silky from the eggs, sweet and salty from the bacon and shallots, and just about everything you want out of breakfast.

5 strips all-natural bacon, diced
1 cup thinly sliced shallots
3 cups finely chopped packed kale
8 eggs
⅓ cup unsweetened almond milk
¼ teaspoon black pepper
¼ teaspoon crushed red pepper
Serve with fresh salsa

> **NOTE:** It is so important to buy quality bacon from pigs who are responsibly raised. Factory-farmed pigs are raised in horrible, overcrowded living conditions, not fed their natural diets, given additives and anti-biotics, which in turn cause numerous health conditions and lead to a build-up of toxins in the pigs. Whenever I purchase bacon I make sure it is free of nitrates, humanely and sustainably-farmed and sugar-free.

1. Pre-heat your oven to 375 degrees.

2. In a non-stick oven-safe skillet or cast iron pan, cook your diced bacon until crispy. Remove the bacon from the skillet and render the fat. Add the shallots to the skillet and sauté them about 5 minutes or until they are nicely browned and begin to get crispy. Remove the shallots from the skillet then add in the kale and sauté for 2 minutes or until it is withered. Remove from the skillet and set aside.

3. In a large bowl, mix together the eggs, almond milk, and peppers. Turn the heat to low and spray the skillet with a non-stick cooking spray. Add the egg mixture to the skillet then add in the withered kale and cooked bacon. Gently mix everything together making sure the frittata is even on all sides. Let the eggs cook and set on low heat in the skillet for about 5 minutes (do not sauté the eggs or you will end up with a scramble). Top the frittata with the crispy shallots then place the skillet in the oven. Bake the frittata for 12–15 minutes or until the eggs are cooked through. Remove the skillet from the oven, slice the frittata into equal pieces and serve immediately.

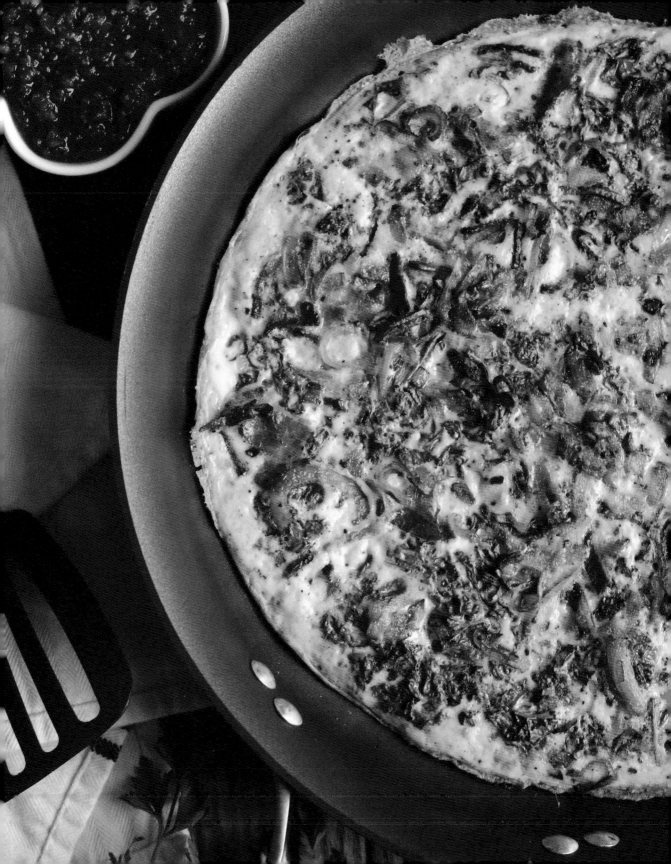

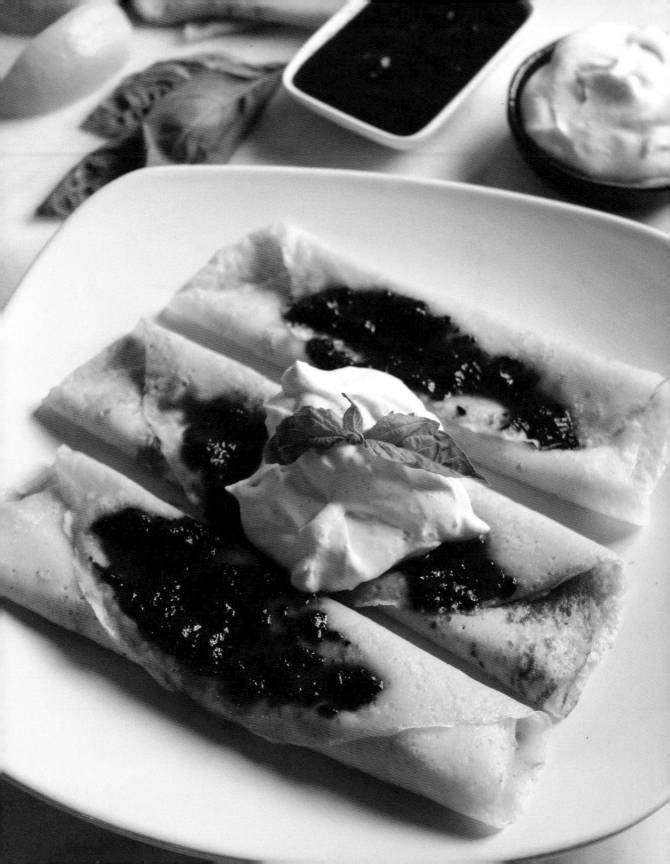

CREPES WITH BLUEBERRY-BASIL SAUCE AND COCONUT WHIPPED CREAM

Gluten-Free, Dairy-Free, Vegetarian

Yields 8–10 Crepes

These crepes come out so perfectly thin and pair wonderfully with the blueberry-basil sauce. The best part is the coconut whipped cream. You literally can't taste the difference between this and dairy whipped cream! And PS try a dollop of this coconut whipped cream recipe in your coffee next time—it's a life changer.

Crepe Batter:
1½ cups almond milk
2 eggs
1½ tablespoons honey
1 tablespoon coconut oil
¼ teaspoon salt
1 cup gluten-free all-purpose flour
   (Bob's Red Mill Gluten-Free
   All-Purpose Flour works great)

Blueberry-Basil Sauce:
1 cup fresh blueberries
1 tablespoon lemon juice
1 tablespoon + 1 teaspoon honey
1 tablespoon roughly chopped
   packed basil

Coconut Whipped Cream:
1 (13.5-ounce) can full-fat coconut
   milk (placed in the refrigerator
   for at least 12 hours)
2 teaspoons honey
¼ teaspoon cinnamon

1. In a large bowl, mix together the almond milk, eggs, honey, coconut oil, and salt. Using an electric hand mixer, slowly add in the flour. Mix until the batter is well combined and there are no clumps. Cover the bowl and place in the refrigerator.

2. For the cinnamon-coconut whipped cream, place a metal or steel bowl in the freezer for 10 minutes. After 10 minutes, remove the bowl from the freezer. Scoop just the cream that forms at the top of the can of coconut milk into the bowl. This cream can be thicker sometimes, so if this is the case just add in a few teaspoons of the coconut water at the bottom of the can to thin it out. Add in the honey and cinnamon, then using an electric hand mixer, blend the cream on high for 3–5 minutes or until firm peaks begin to form. Cover the bowl and place it in the refrigerator until ready to use.

3. To make the blueberry-basil sauce, place all ingredients in a food processor and process until the sauce is completely smooth. Transfer the sauce to a bowl and set aside.

4. To make the crepes, heat a small non-stick skillet. Once the skillet is heated, keep it on a medium-low heat. Grease the pan with a non-stick cooking spray and ladle the batter to the center of the pan. Swirl the pan to spread the batter out thin and evenly. Cook the crepe for 30 seconds then gently flip it and cook the other side for 10–15 seconds. Make sure to grease the pan for each crepe. Serve the crepes rolled, topped with the blueberry sauce and a dollop of the cinnamon-coconut whipped cream.

HASH BROWN AND EGG CUPS

Gluten-Free, Dairy-Free, Grain-Free, Vegetarian

Makes 5 Cups

These little hash brown and egg cups are not only adorable, but the perfect for on-the-go! I love making these early in the week then heating them up in the morning for a quick, yet scrumptious breakfast.

3 cups grated russet potatoes
½ teaspoon salt
5 eggs
½ teaspoon thyme
¼ teaspoon crushed red pepper
Dash of black pepper

Serve with ketchup or hot sauce

1. Preheat your oven to 425 degrees.

2. First, peel your potatoes then grate them. Squeeze out the excess moisture from the grated potatoes.

3. Grease a muffin pan then place the grated potatoes in the muffin slots and gently press the potatoes down creating a cup. Sprinkle the potatoes with ¼ teaspoon of salt. Bake the potatoes for about 15 minutes then remove them from the oven.

4. Crack each egg into the hash brown cups. Sprinkle the tops of the eggs with the remaining ¼ teaspoon of salt, thyme, crushed red pepper, and black pepper. Return to the oven and bake for 10–15 minutes depending on how runny you prefer your yolk.

5. Remove the pan from the oven and gently remove each cup. Serve the hash brown and egg cups dipped in ketchup or hot sauce.

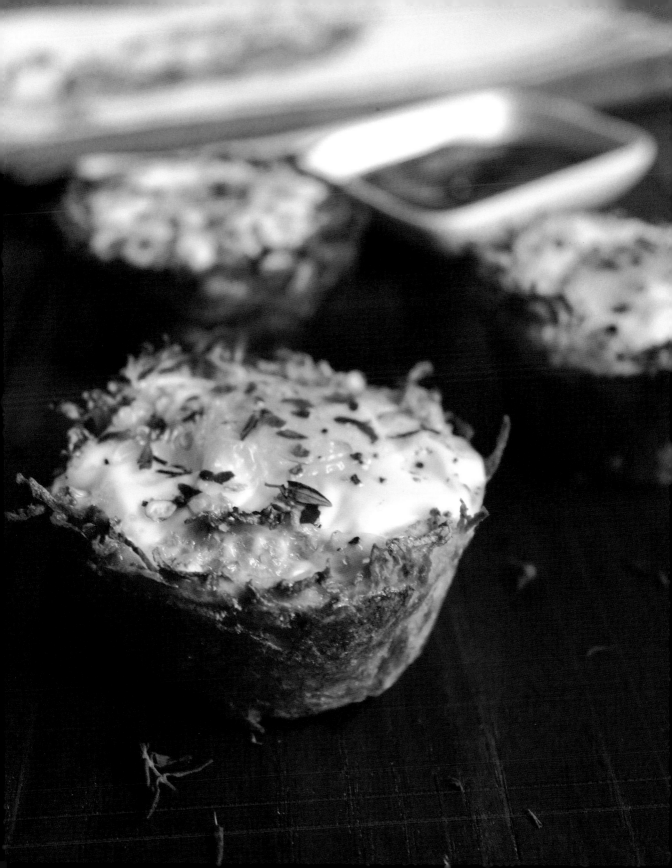

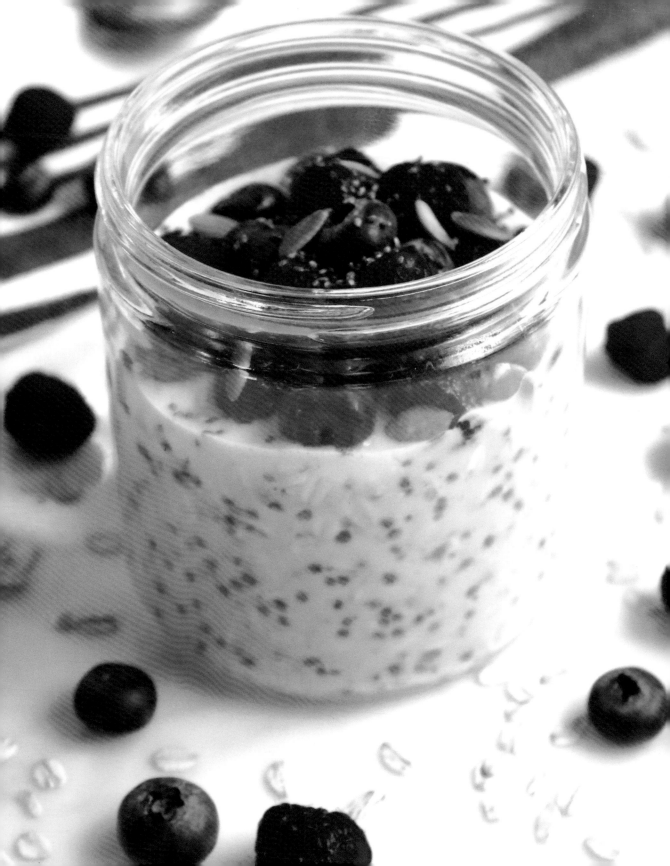

OVERNIGHT OATS

Gluten-Free, Dairy-Free, Vegetarian

Single Serving

Overnight oats are the single most easy breakfast on the planet. You prepare the oats the night before so when you wake up, your breakfast is ready! We prefer the oats served cold, topped with fresh fruit, but you can heat up the oats in the morning if you feel like something warm and comforting.

½ cup rolled oats
1 cup almond milk
1 tablespoon honey
2 teaspoons chia seeds
¼ teaspoon cinnamon
Dash of nutmeg

Toppings:
Fresh raspberries and blueberries
Pumpkin seeds
Additional chia seeds

1. In a mason jar or airtight sealed container, mix together the rolled oats, almond milk, honey, chia seeds, cinnamon, and nutmeg. Place a lid on the jar and leave the oats in the refrigerator overnight, or at least 8 hours.

2. The next morning, remove the overnight oats from the refrigerator and mix everything together again. Top the oats with the berries and seeds.

> *TIP:* When purchasing rolled oats from the grocery store, it's important to buy packages labeled gluten-free. Rolled oats are always naturally gluten-free, however most oats are processed in facilities that also process wheat and therefore could be contaminated with gluten.

BREAKFAST PIZZA

Gluten-Free, Dairy-Free

1–2 Servings

Is there anything better than pizza for breakfast? I think not. This pizza has so many flavors and textures, from the sweet and crispy shallots, the creamy avocado, and the Italian chicken sausage. This recipe could serve one really hungry person, but I prefer to split it with Jason served with a side of fruit or a fresh juice.

*8-inch pre-made gluten-free
   pizza crust*
2 teaspoons extra-virgin olive oil
*⅓ cup sweet Italian chicken
   sausage*
⅓ cup thinly sliced shallots
1 egg
½ avocado, smashed
3 slices tomatoes
*1 tablespoon roughly chopped
   fresh basil*
Salt, to taste
Pinch of crushed red pepper

> **TIP:** For this recipe, I use the Rustic Pizza Gluten-Free Crust. It's all-natural with non-GMO ingredients. If you don't feel like making your own pizza dough, this pre-made crust works in a pinch!

1. Preheat your oven to 450 degrees. Brush the pizza crust with 1 teaspoon olive oil and bake it according to the instructions on the package.

2. In a skillet, cook your chicken sausage. Once the sausage is cooked and crumbled, transfer it to a bowl and cover with foil so the sausage stays warm. Add 1 teaspoon olive oil and the shallots to the skillet, sautéing them a few minutes, or until the shallots become browned and start to get crispy. Transfer to a bowl and cover. In the same skillet, crack the egg and fry it according to how runny you prefer the yolk.

3. Remove the pizza crust from the oven once it's done baking and allow it to cool. Once cooled, spread the smashed avocado on the crust then top it with the tomato slices, crumbled sausage, fried egg, shallots, basil, salt, and crushed red pepper. Slice the pizza four ways and serve.

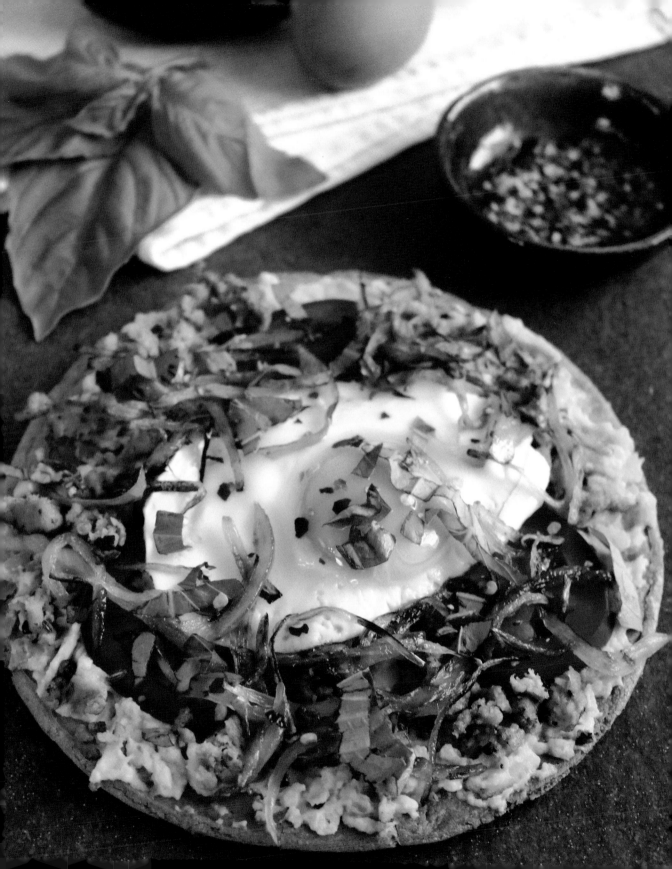

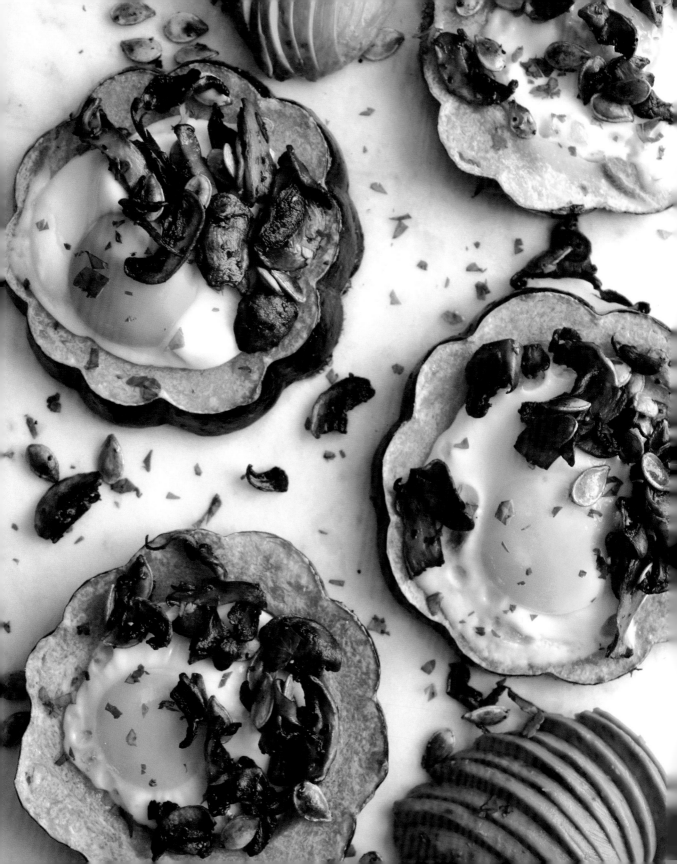

BAKED EGGS IN ACORN SQUASH

Gluten-Free, Dairy-Free, Grain-Free, Vegetarian

Makes 4 Egg Rings

So, not only are these so pretty to look at, but they are super tasty. I love the sweet, buttery texture of the roasted acorn squash combined with the richness of the egg yolk, then the salty earthiness you get from the mushrooms and pumpkin seeds.

4 acorn squash slices, cut into ½ inch pieces, seeds and core removed
1 tablespoon extra-virgin olive oil
4 eggs
⅛ teaspoon salt
Black pepper, to taste

Toppings:

2 cups thinly sliced white mushrooms
2 tablespoons pumpkin seeds
1 tablespoon extra-virgin olive oil
¼ teaspoon salt
¼ teaspoon black pepper
Fresh minced Italian parsley, to top

Serve with avocado slices

1. Preheat your oven to 425 degrees.

2. Brush the top and bottom of each acorn squash slice in olive oil. Place the acorn squash slices on a baking sheet and bake them for 15 minutes, then remove the baking pan from the oven. Spray the center of the squash slices with a nonstick cooking spray or grease with oil. Crack an egg into the center of each squash slice. Sprinkle with salt and black pepper then return the baking sheet to the oven. Bake for 6–10 minutes (6 minutes for over easy, 10 minutes for over hard).

3. In a skillet, sauté the mushrooms and pumpkin seeds in 1 tablespoon of olive oil until the pumpkin seeds are roasted and the mushrooms are browned and crispy, about 6–8 minutes. Season the mushrooms and pumpkin seeds with salt and pepper.

4. Serve the baked eggs in acorn squash topped with the mushrooms and pumpkin seeds, minced parsley, and avocado slices.

FACT: You can eat the skin of the roasted acorn squash! It contains many nutrients and has a great texture.

SWEET POTATO BREAKFAST SLIDERS

Gluten-Free, Dairy-Free, Grain-Free

Single Serving (3 Sliders)

Sometimes I get sick of always making eggs for breakfast, so I come back to these! The baked sweet potatoes are the perfect replacement for buns and they are a whole new, amazing take on traditional sliders.

*6 sweet potato slices, sliced about
    ¼ inch thick*
2 teaspoons coconut oil
½ avocado, smashed
Pinch of salt
3 slices tomato
3 slices deli-style turkey meat

1. Preheat your oven to 425 degrees.

2. Brush each side of your sweet potato slices in coconut oil. Place the sweet potatoes on a foil-lined baking sheet and bake for 15–20 minutes, flipping halfway through. Once the sweet potatoes are cooked, remove them from the oven and allow them to cool.

3. In a small bowl, combine the avocado and salt.

4. To assemble the sliders: Spread the avocado on a baked sweet potato slice, top with the tomato and turkey meat, then spread more avocado on the bottom of another baked sweet potato slice and place it on top. Repeat these steps for the next two sliders. Serve immediately.

> *TIP:* My favorite brand of store-bought turkey meat is Plainville Farms. It's so hard to come across an organic, deli-style turkey meat that isn't filled with preservatives and sugar, and this one is not only delicious, but has three total ingredients: organic turkey, salt, and water.

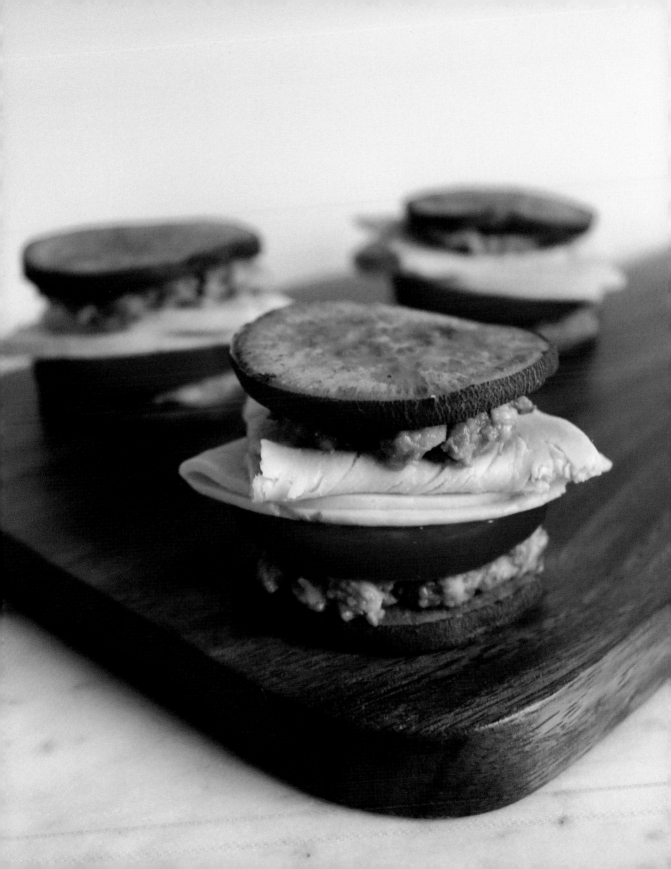

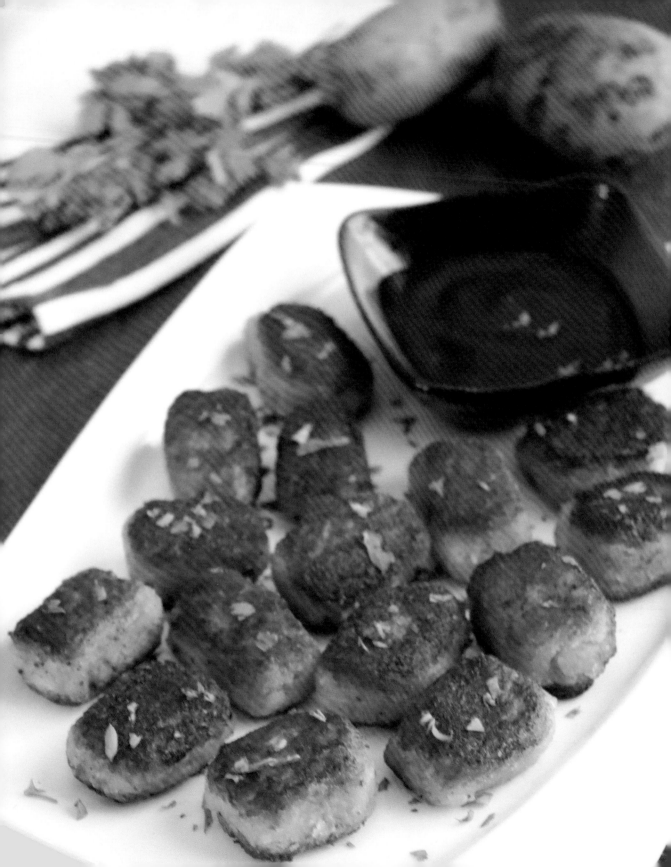

TATER-TOTS

Gluten-Free, Dairy-Free, Vegan

Makes about 16 Tots

When you hear "tater-tots," the word "healthy" doesn't always come to mind. That's because traditional store-bought tater-tots are filled with additives, chemicals, and preservatives, and typically don't even contain much potato! This recipe is so simple to make, crispy on the outside, and super creamy on the inside—it's going to leave you wondering where this recipe has been all your life.

2 large russet potatoes, peeled and washed
½ tablespoon gluten-free all-purpose flour
½ teaspoon salt
½ teaspoon garlic powder
½ teaspoon onion powder
¼ teaspoon paprika
¼ teaspoon black pepper
4 tablespoons coconut oil
Fresh minced parsley, to top

Serve with ketchup for dipping

1. Bring a small pot of water to a boil, then add in the peeled, whole potatoes. Par-boil the potatoes for about 12 minutes. You don't want to overcook them, as they still need to be firm enough to grate. Drain the potatoes then let them cool for about 5 minutes.

2. Once the potatoes have cooled, grate them into a medium-sized bowl. Once grated, add in the flour and all seasonings (except parsley). Combine all ingredients well with your hands.

3. Form 1-inch tater-tots by molding them with your hands into a cylinder shape. If your hands get sticky from the potato starch, rinse them with water and keep going.

4. Heat a skillet on medium heat with the coconut oil. Add the tater-tots to the skillet, being careful not to overcrowd them. Fry each side for 4–5 minutes or until nicely browned and crispy.

5. Serve the tater-tots topped with minced parsley, additional salt if desired, and a side of ketchup for dipping.

POACHED EGGS WITH VEGETABLE HASH

Gluten-Free, Dairy-Free, Grain-Free, Vegetarian

2 Servings

Who doesn't love a poached egg? They are so creamy and delectable, not to mention pretty. After watching a few videos on the internet, I mastered the art of poaching eggs, and I am here to show you how easy it is! The poached egg over vegetable hash topped with avocado truly makes for the perfect, simple, and utterly delicious breakfast.

2 tablespoons coconut oil
1 cup thinly sliced yellow onions
1 cup thinly sliced red bell peppers
2 cups Brussels sprouts, trimmed and thinly sliced
2 cups chopped white mushrooms
2 garlic cloves, minced
½ teaspoon salt
½ teaspoon black pepper
2 eggs
Dash of apple cider vinegar
1 avocado, sliced
Fresh Italian parsley, minced, to top

1. For the vegetable hash, heat 1 tablespoon of coconut oil in a skillet. Add in the onions and bell peppers and sauté for about 5 minutes, or until the onions are translucent and the bell peppers are softened. Now add in the other 1 tablespoon of coconut oil, Brussels sprouts, and mushrooms. Continue to sauté the vegetables a few minutes, then lastly add in the garlic, salt, and pepper. Sauté the hash until the vegetables are nicely browned, about 5 more minutes.

2. For the poached eggs, fill about ⅔ of a medium-sized saucepan with water, then bring the water to a boil. Once the water is boiling, reduce the heat so the water can relax and simmer. Crack each egg into an individual, small ramekin cup. Throw a few dashes of apple cider vinegar into the simmering water. Using the ramekin cup, carefully and gently lower then tip each egg into the water. Set your timer for 4–6 minutes (depending on how runny you prefer the yolk). Use a slotted spoon to remove each egg from the water and place them on a paper towel. If there are any wispy egg whites around the egg, just cut them off.

3. Spoon the vegetable hash into a shallow bowl then top it with the poached egg, sliced avocado, and minced parsley. You may also add additional salt and black pepper to top.

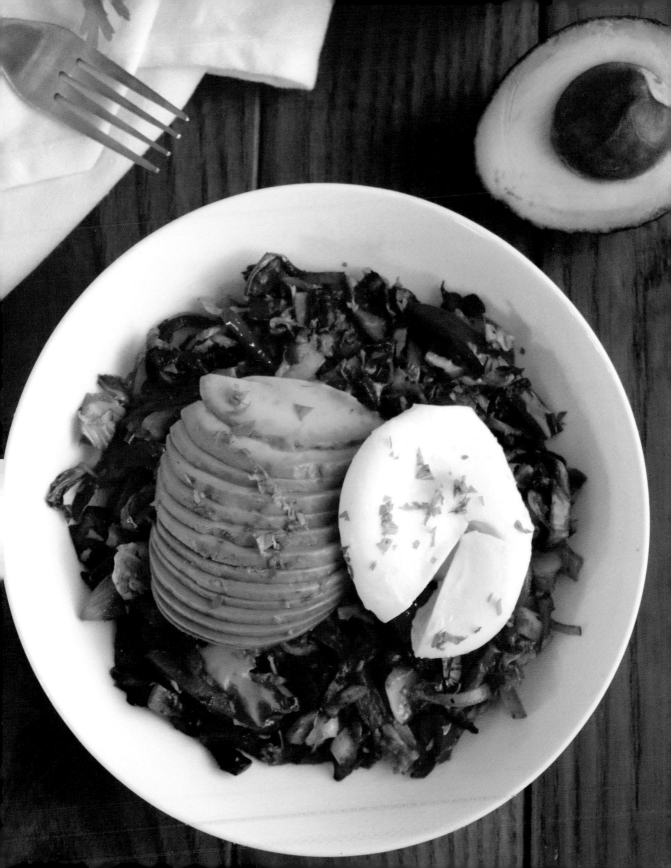

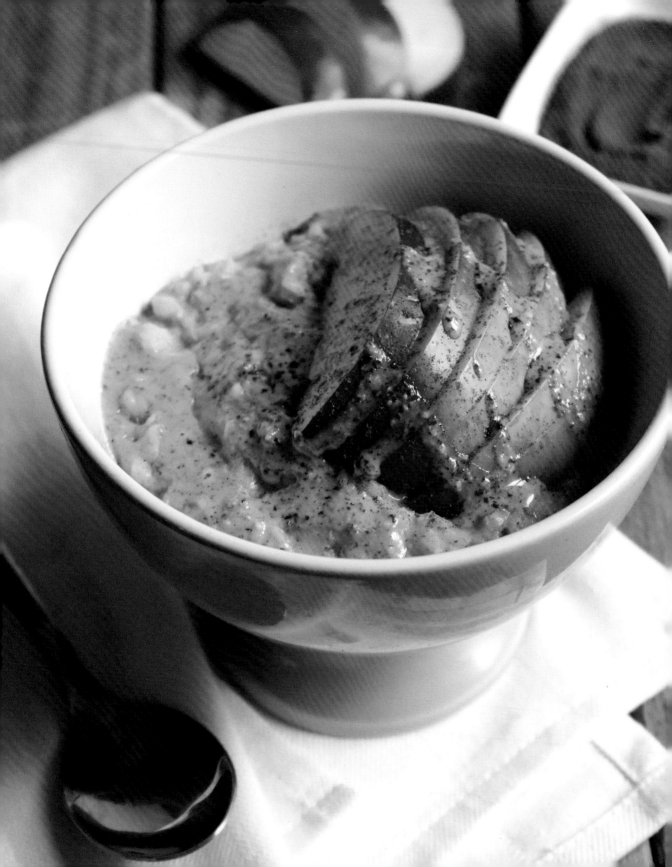

APPLE-CINNAMON OATMEAL WITH ALMOND-COCONUT DRIZZLE

Gluten-Free, Dairy-Free, Vegetarian

Single Serving

If you love apple pie, then you will love this recipe. It's warm, cozy, and makes for an irresistible breakfast.

1½ cups almond milk
½ cup rolled oats
¼ cup unsweetened applesauce
2 teaspoons honey
¼ teaspoon salt
¼ teaspoon cinnamon

Almond-Coconut Drizzle:
2 teaspoons almond butter
1 teaspoon coconut oil

Apple slices and additional
    cinnamon, to top

1. In a medium-sized saucepan, bring the almond milk to a boil. Add in the rolled oats then turn the heat to low and let the oatmeal cook 10–15 minutes or until the almond milk is absorbed, stirring the oatmeal every so often. Now add in the applesauce, honey, salt, and cinnamon.

2. In a small bowl, mix together the almond butter and coconut oil.

3. Transfer the oatmeal to a bowl and top with fresh apple slices, the almond-coconut drizzle, and a pinch of cinnamon.

> *FACT:* Oats are loaded in dietary fiber, have a range of cholesterol-lowering properties, and have been shown to help reduce the risk of heart disease.

ROSEMARY-NUTMEG SCOTCH EGGS

Gluten-Free, Dairy-Free, Grain-Free

2 Servings

Traditional Scotch Eggs are made with some type of pork sausage and rolled in bread crumbs then deep fried, but in my rendition, I use ground beef with an almond meal crust and bake them. I love the aroma of the nutmeg and rosemary while these beauties bake. Jason can't get enough of these every time I make this recipe! Scotch eggs are high in protein and good fat to keep you fueled and energized throughout the day.

4 eggs
½ pound ground beef
1 teaspoon minced rosemary
¼ teaspoon nutmeg
½ teaspoon garlic powder
½ teaspoon onion powder
¼ teaspoon salt
¼ teaspoon black pepper
¼ teaspoon crushed red pepper

Almond Meal Crust:

1 egg
¼ cup unsweetened almond milk
⅓ cup almond meal
Dash of salt

1. Preheat the oven to 425 degrees.

2. Boil your eggs anywhere from 4–12 minutes, depending on how you prefer the yolk. We prefer our eggs hard-boiled for this recipe. Allow the eggs to cool, then peel them and set aside.

3. Combine the ground beef and seasonings in a bowl. Separate the seasoned beef into four equal parts. In a separate bowl, combine the egg and almond milk. In another bowl, combine the almond meal and salt. Take the beef and smash it down like a pancake then take the boiled egg and mold the beef around the egg making sure no egg white is showing through.

4. Dip each covered egg in the egg wash, then roll it in the almond meal until completely covered.

5. Grease a baking sheet and place each Scotch egg on the sheet. Bake for 25–30 minutes or until the outer crust is browned and the beef is cooked through. Remove from the oven and let them cool for 5 minutes.

6. Slice each egg in half then sprinkle each half with additional salt and hot sauce.

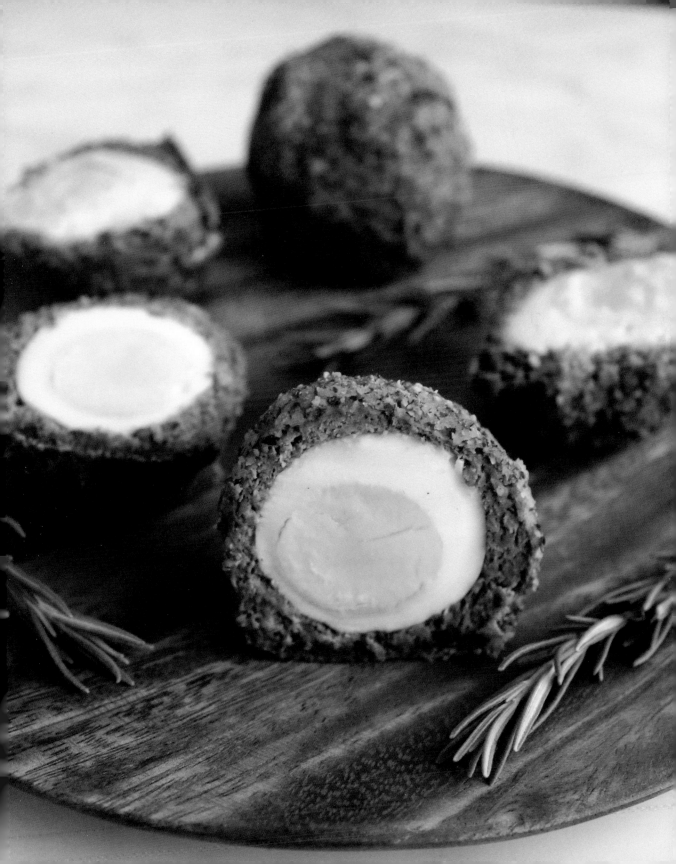

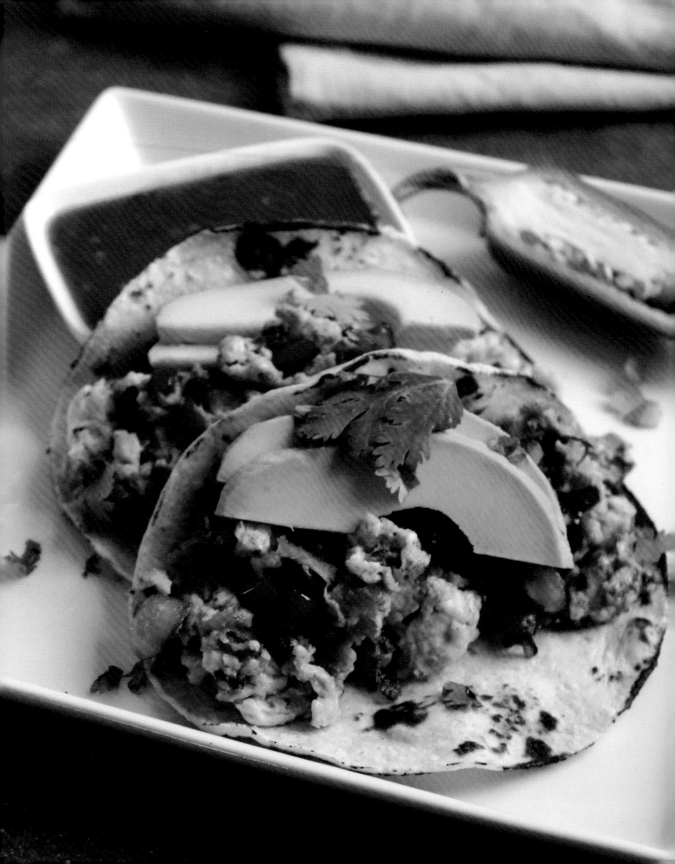

BREAKFAST TACOS

Gluten-Free, Dairy-Free

2 Servings (Makes 4 Large Tacos)

Any morning can immediately be made better with breakfast tacos. If Jason could have these tacos every morning, he absolutely would. The filling for the tacos has so much intense flavor and is perfectly complemented by the warm corn tortillas, avocado slices, and fresh cilantro.

2 slices all-natural bacon, diced
½ cup diced red bell pepper
⅓ cup minced yellow onion
1 tablespoon minced jalapeño
½ tablespoon olive oil
4 eggs
Dash of salt
4 corn tortillas

Toppings:

1 small avocado, sliced
Fresh cilantro, minced

Serve with fresh salsa

> **NOTE:** Most corn tortillas are gluten-free, however I have come across brands that add in wheat flour, so always check your ingredients labels. Also, try to always buy organic corn tortillas as most corn that is produced in the United States comes from GMO crops.

1. In a skillet, sauté the bacon until it becomes crispy. Remove the bacon from the skillet and render the bacon fat. Now add in the red bell peppers, onion, jalapeño, and olive oil. Sauté until the onions are translucent and the bell peppers and jalapeños begin to soften. Add the bacon back into the skillet along with the eggs. Mix everything together and continue to sauté for about a minute or until the eggs are cooked through. Top with a dash of salt and turn off the heat.

2. Warm each corn tortilla on a burner 10–15 seconds per side. Fill the tortillas with the egg filling, then top each taco with avocado slices, cilantro, and serve with fresh salsa.

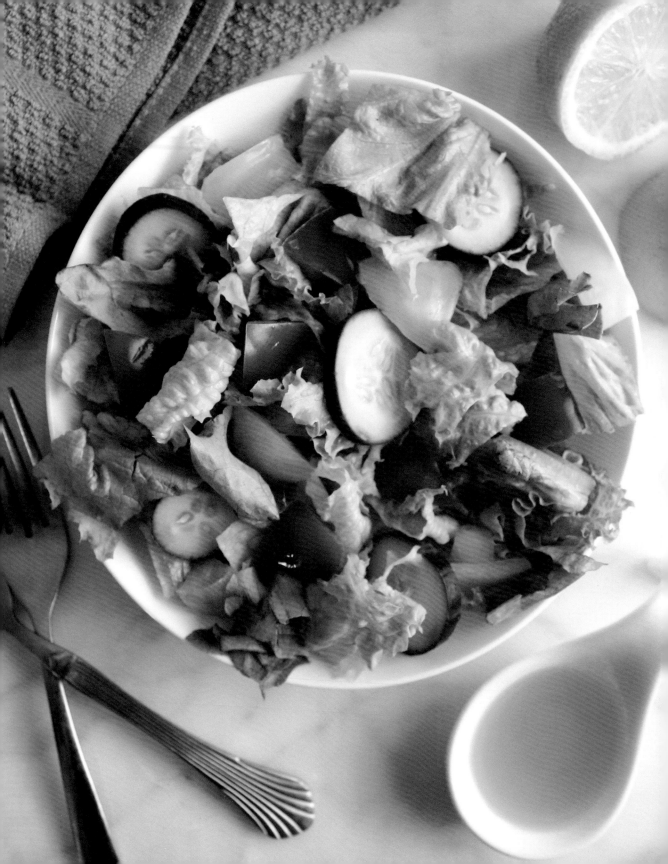

Lunch, Small Bites, and Appetizers

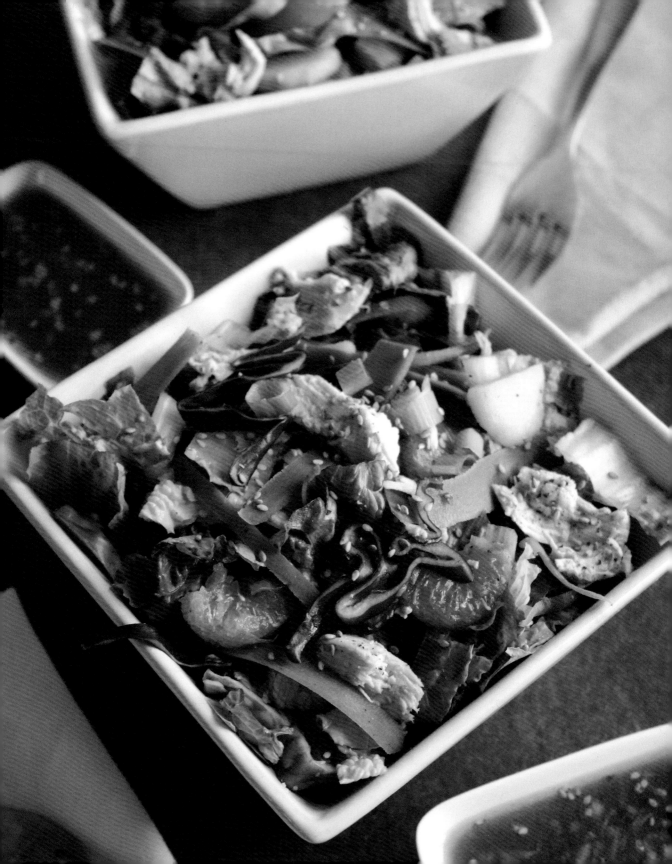

CHINESE CHICKEN SALAD WITH SESAME-GINGER DRESSING

Gluten-Free, Dairy-Free, Grain-Free

3–4 Servings

If there is a Chinese chicken salad on the menu at any restaurant, I'm ordering it. I love the components of this classic salad: the textures, the crunch, the tanginess from the dressing. So I wanted to create a version that anyone can make at home with little effort, and still end up with a restaurant-quality salad. Mission accomplished!

6 cups chopped romaine lettuce
2 cups shredded cooked chicken
3 cups shredded purple cabbage
1 cup Mandarin orange slices
½ cup water chestnuts, sliced in halves
1 cup shredded carrots
½ cup chopped green onions
⅓ cup almond slivers
½ cup sugar snap peas
½ teaspoon black pepper
Sesame seeds, to top

Sesame-Ginger Dressing:
½ cup apple cider vinegar
1 tablespoon sesame oil
2 tablespoons honey
2 tablespoons coconut aminos
1 tablespoon coconut oil
½ teaspoon sesame seeds
1 teaspoon grated ginger
½ teaspoon of grated garlic

1. In a large bowl, toss together all salad ingredients until thoroughly combined.

2. In a separate small bowl or mason jar, mix together all salad dressing ingredients. Serve the salad drizzled in the dressing.

> **TIP:** To easily grate ginger, peel the outer skin using a potato peeler, then use a box grater.

VEGETARIAN PORTOBELLO MUSHROOM PIZZAS

Gluten-Free, Dairy-Free, Grain-Free, Vegan

Makes 4 Mini Pizzas

The Portobello mushrooms act as the pizza crust, and once baked, they have this wonderful, meaty texture. The vegetables that top the pizza, accompanied by the fresh tomato sauce, are really the perfect combination. You can also add any type of meat in addition to the vegetables if you want, such as a nice Italian sausage. I love to serve these savory little pizzas as an appetizer for a small dinner party.

4 large Portobello mushroom caps
2 tablespoons extra-virgin olive oil
½ teaspoon salt
½ cup tomato sauce (recipe on page 116)
⅓ cup thinly sliced red onion
⅓ cup diced yellow bell pepper
½–1 thinly sliced jalapeño (depending on how spicy you like it)
2 asparagus spears, cut in fourths
2 garlic cloves, minced
⅓ cup roughly chopped fresh basil

1. Preheat the oven to 425 degrees.

2. For the Portobello mushrooms, first remove the stem, then the black gills. To remove the gills, start from the center of the mushroom and scoop them out with a spoon. These mushrooms can be fragile and can break, so scoop gently. I like to cut around the edges of the mushrooms caps so they are perfectly circular. Brush the tops and bottoms of the mushrooms in the olive oil then sprinkle with salt.

3. On a foil-lined baking sheet, bake the mushrooms for 8 minutes then remove from the oven. If liquid forms in the mushroom caps, just soak it up with a paper towel. Top the mushrooms with the tomato sauce, onions, bell peppers, jalapeños, and asparagus. Place them back in the oven and bake for 10–12 more minutes, then sprinkle the garlic on top and bake another 5 minutes (you don't want the garlic to burn).

4. Remove the pizzas from the oven and allow then to cool a few minutes. Serve them topped with the fresh basil.

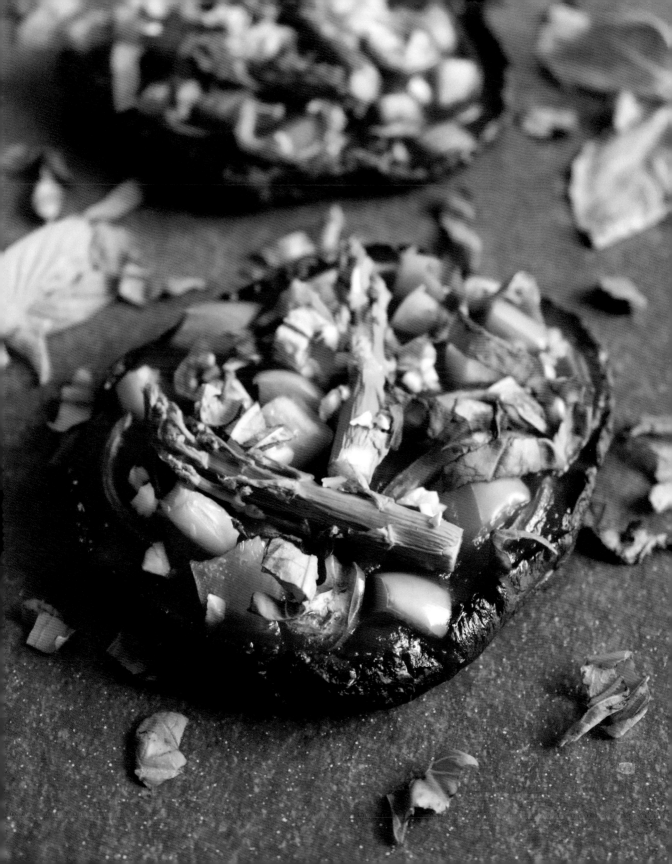

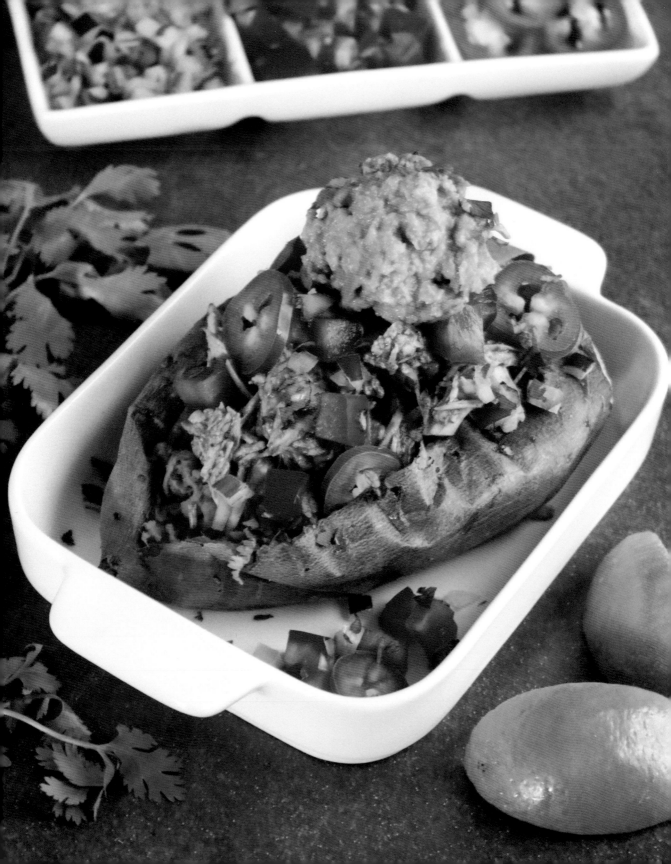

TEX-MEX FILLED SWEET POTATOES

Gluten-Free, Dairy-Free, Grain-Free

2 Servings

This has been one of my most popular and re-posted recipes on Instagram—and for good reason! Not only is this recipe absolutely scrumptious, but it's so easy to put together for a quick lunch, or even dinner. The flavors and textures blend perfectly, and the beautiful colors make it exciting to dig your fork into.

2 small sweet potatoes
1 cup shredded cooked chicken
2 tablespoons barbeque sauce
Dash of salt and black pepper

Toppings:
½ cup diced tomatoes
2 tablespoons minced red onions
1 avocado, smashed
1 small jalapeño, sliced thin
2 teaspoons minced cilantro

1. Preheat the oven to 425 degrees. Poke holes on the tops of the sweet potatoes and place them on a foil-lined baking sheet. Bake the sweet potatoes for 45–60 minutes, depending on the size.

2. In a small bowl, mix together the cooked chicken, barbeque sauce, and seasonings, and set aside. Once the sweet potatoes are cooked, remove them from the oven and slice them lengthwise through the middle, but not completely through. Stuff the potatoes with the barbeque chicken mixture and return them to the oven for 5–8 minutes or until the chicken is hot. Remove the potatoes from the oven, then top with the tomatoes, onions, avocado, jalapeño slices, and cilantro.

3. Serve with additional barbeque sauce as desired.

RAINBOW SPRING ROLLS WITH SHRIMP

Gluten-Free, Dairy-Free

Makes 20 Spring Rolls

These spring rolls are a great, refreshing, summertime appetizer, and are completely gorgeous from all the different colors in the filling. Spring rolls are one of our favorite things to order whenever we eat Vietnamese food, and I've been making these now for years. The technique of rolling them can be a bit difficult at first, but once you get it down, it's so easy.

20 sheets of rice paper (these can be found at any grocery store in the Asian section)
20 medium-sized shrimp, cooked and sliced in halves
2–3 avocados, sliced thin
2 red mangos, julienned
3 cups shredded purple cabbage
2 large carrots, julienned
1 large cucumber, julienned
5 cups shredded green leaf lettuce

Serve with creamy peanut sauce (recipe on page 123)

1. First, make sure all the vegetables and fruit are cut, then create an assembly line to easily roll the spring rolls.

2. Fill a large bowl with warm water. Place each piece of rice paper in the warm water for about 15 seconds, until it becomes pliable. Lay the wet rice paper on a dry, non-porous surface. On one side of the rice paper, add in the shrimp, avocado, mango, cabbage, carrots, cucumber, and a bit of lettuce, keeping at least a few inches open at each edge so they easily roll (it's much harder to roll these if they are overstuffed). Once the rice paper feels sticky and not wet, fold in the edges of the rice paper and roll. As you're rolling them, make sure you tuck the fillings together so they don't fall out and roll the spring rolls as tightly as possible (if this doesn't make sense, there are plenty of YouTube videos out there that show you exactly how this is done).

3. Serve the spring rolls with the creamy peanut sauce for dipping.

NOTE: This recipe makes a large quantity suited for an appetizer. If you cut the recipe in half, it will serve 2–3 people.

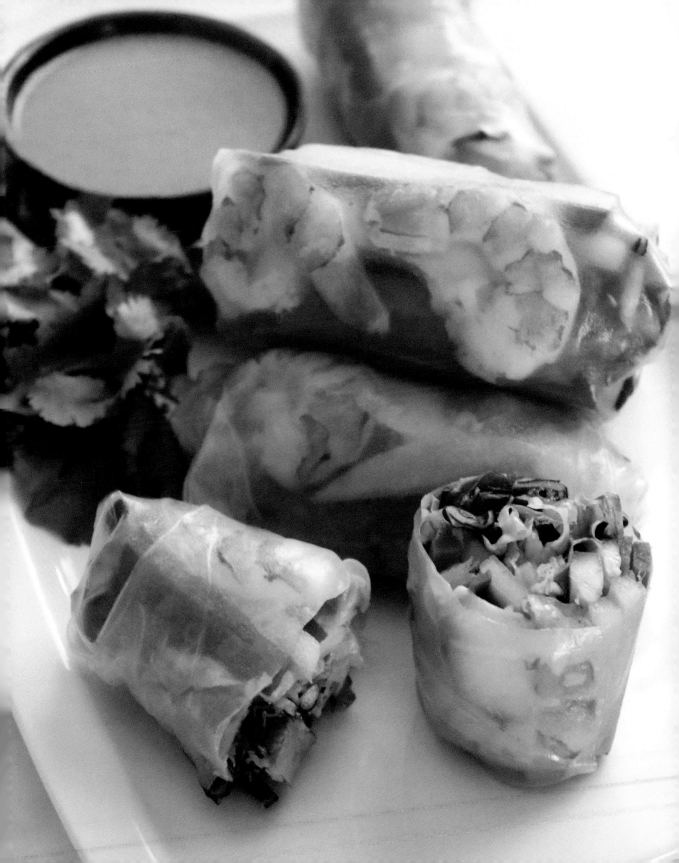

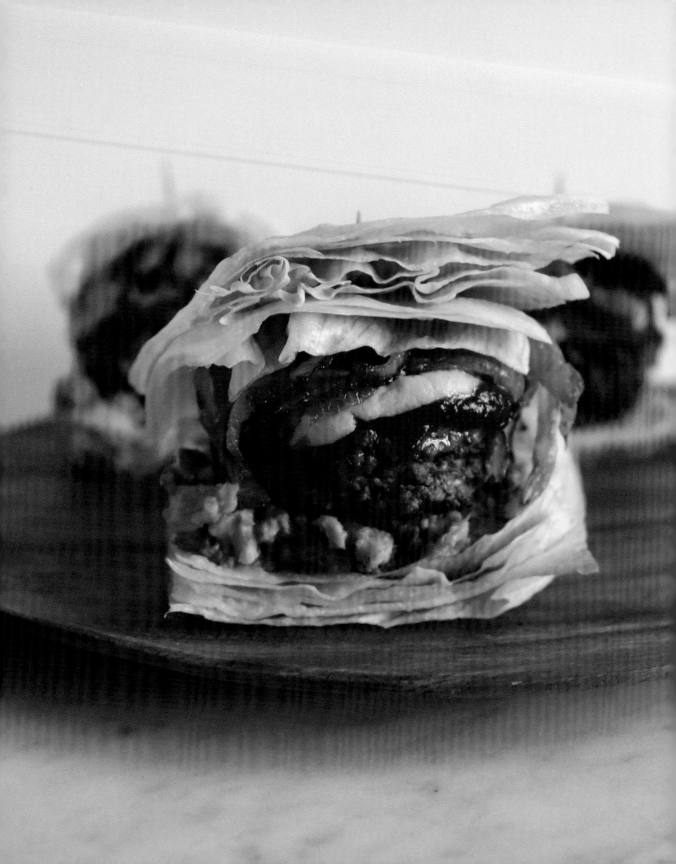

LETTUCE-WRAPPED BEEF SLIDERS

Gluten-Free, Dairy-Free, Grain-Free

Makes 6 Sliders (2–3 Servings)

Jason and I have always been fans of hamburgers (who isn't, right?), so when we went gluten-free, I feared it would be difficult to give up those buns. Turns out, we actually like our burgers wrapped in lettuce better! You get to taste the flavors of the juicy patty and the delicious toppings, as opposed to everything being soaked up in the bread. You are also left feeling light and not overly-stuffed. These sliders are so flavorful I promise you won't miss the bread.

¾ pound ground beef, shaped into 6 balls
Salt and pepper, as desired

Toppings:
2 cups thinly sliced onions
1 tablespoon extra-virgin olive oil
1 large head iceberg lettuce
2 small avocados, smashed
9 cherry tomatoes, sliced in half

Drizzle the sliders in ketchup and yellow mustard as desired

1. In a skillet, sauté your onions in olive oil until nicely browned, set aside.

2. Season each side of the burger patties well with salt and pepper. Grill your burger patties by smashing them down and grilling each side 3–4 minutes.

3. Slice the bottom core off the head of iceberg lettuce. Slice the head in half, then slice each half three ways. You can trim the lettuce pieces to be more square so they are nice and pretty.

4. To assemble the sliders, take a few pieces from the sliced iceberg lettuce and spread some avocado then top with the beef patty, ketchup, mustard, cherry tomatoes, grilled onions, then a few more pieces of the iceberg lettuce. Secure everything with a toothpick and serve immediately.

MANGO HABANERO BAKED CHICKEN WINGS

Gluten-Free, Dairy-Free, Grain-Free

Makes 15 Wings (2–3 Servings)

We love the mango habanero flavor at Buffalo Wild Wings, but when I looked up the sauce ingredients online, I realized I needed to come up with my own clean version of this recipe. This mango-habanero sauce is a perfect balance of sweet and spicy, and the wings actually get really crispy when oven-baked. The secret to crispy oven-baked wings? A cooling rack! It allows the juices from the chicken to drip onto the pan below instead of soaking into the skin and making it soggy while they bake.

1 teaspoon salt
1 teaspoon garlic powder
½ teaspoon paprika
2 pounds chicken wings
  (about 15 pieces)

Mango Habanero Sauce:
1 cup diced mango
2 habanero peppers, sliced in half
  (for mild-hot spice)
1 cup roughly chopped yellow
  onion
2 large garlic cloves
3 large pitted dates
½ cup apple cider vinegar
2 tablespoons coconut aminos
½ teaspoon salt
½ teaspoon paprika

1. Preheat your oven to 425 degrees. Line a baking sheet with foil, place a cooling rack on top of the baking sheet, and spray the cooling rack with a non-stick cooking spray.

2. In a high-power blender (not a food processor—it doesn't puree the sauce as well), blend all mango habanero ingredients until completely smooth. Transfer to a small saucepan. Bring the sauce to a boil, then reduce the heat to low, cover, and simmer while the wings bake, stirring the sauce every so often.

3. In a small bowl, mix together the salt, garlic powder, and paprika. Place the chicken wings in a large plastic bag with the seasoning, and shake it so all pieces are evenly seasoned. Place the wings on the cooling rack, being careful not to overcrowd them. Bake the wings for 30 minutes, then flip them over and bake an additional 20 minutes or until the outer skin is crispy and the chicken is cooked through.

4. Set the oven to broil. Transfer the mango habanero sauce to a large bowl and toss the baked wings in the sauce until they are evenly coated. Place the wings back on the cooling rack and broil 3–5 minutes until the wings are glazed and crispy. Serve immediately.

NOTE: The mango habanero sauce is initially raw tasting and very spicy, which is why the sauce needs to simmer for at least 30–45 minutes so the flavors can blend and the spices can cook out a bit. If you don't like a lot of spice, I recommend only using 1 habanero pepper.

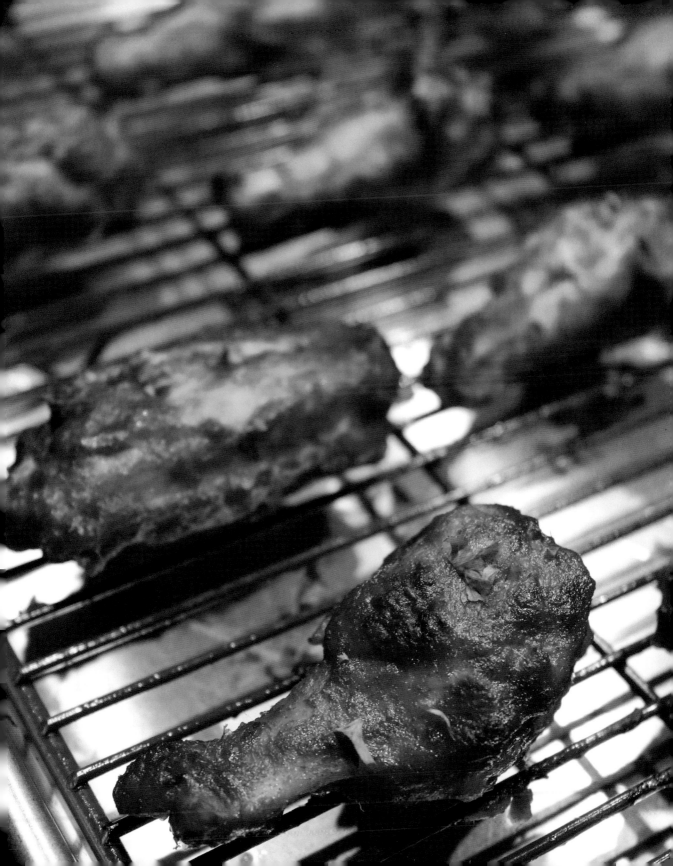

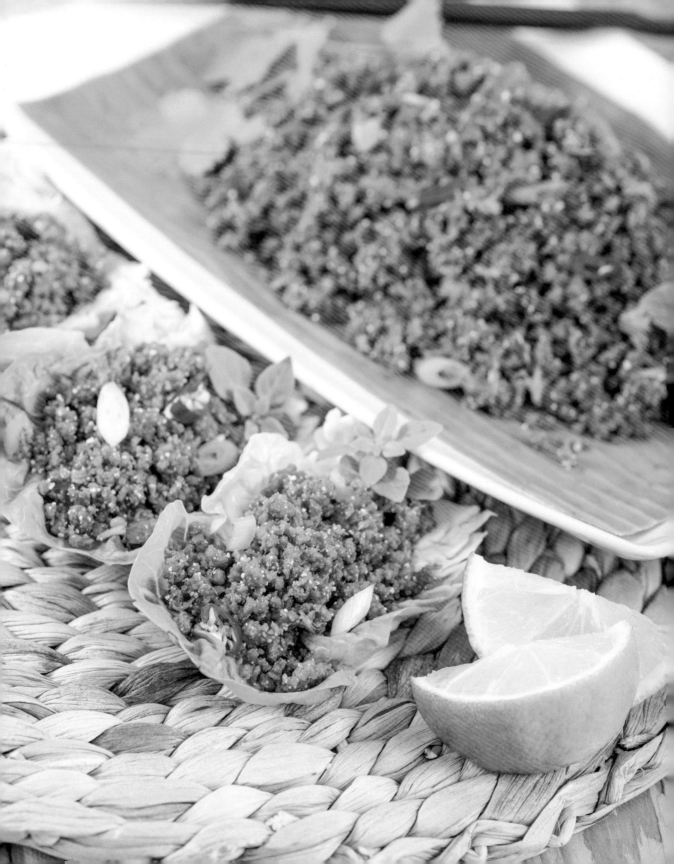

GROUND TURKEY ASIAN LETTUCE WRAPS

Gluten-Free, Dairy-Free, Grain-Free

2–3 Servings

When Jason I first got married and I could barely boil water, let alone *cook* anything (hey, there is hope for all!), this was one of the first recipes I came up with. It's evolved so much over the years and you can really add any type of vegetable into the meat mixture and it will turn out tasting wonderful. This recipe is so filling and I always make plenty for leftovers because it's just as tasty the next day.

½ cup minced yellow onion
1 red bell pepper, diced
1 tablespoon avocado oil
1 pound ground turkey meat
4 garlic cloves, minced
1 cup shredded green cabbage
⅓ cup chopped green onions
1 teaspoon grated fresh ginger
3 tablespoons coconut aminos
1 tablespoon sriracha (recipe on
    page 128)
Dash of salt and black pepper

1 head of iceberg or butterleaf
    lettuce
Serve with creamy peanut sauce
    (recipe on page 123)

1. In a skillet, sauté the onions and bell pepper in avocado oil until the onions are translucent and the bell pepper is softened. Add in the ground turkey and garlic and as the turkey cooks down, break it apart. Then add in the cabbage, green onions, and ginger and sauté a few more minutes until the vegetables and meat are cooked. Now add in the coconut aminos, sriracha, black pepper, and salt. Continue to cook on high heat until all the liquid from the aminos has been absorbed. Transfer to a bowl.

2. Cut the stem off the head of iceberg lettuce then cut it into fourths. Or if you chose to use butterleaf lettuce, just pluck the leaves off the stem and wash them well. Place all the lettuce cups on a plate.

3. To serve, start by using a single lettuce cup, add in the turkey meat mixture, then drizzle with the creamy peanut sauce to top.

> **NOTE:** You will notice I use coconut aminos a lot in my recipes; it's one of my favorite ingredients to add an amazing flavor to any dish. Coconut aminos are made from the nutrient-rich sap that comes out of coconut blossoms when a coconut tree is tapped. It tastes very similar to soy sauce, but has much less sodium, a slightly sweeter taste, and does not taste like coconut at all.

ULTIMATE COBB SALAD WITH CREAMY BALSAMIC DRESSING

Gluten-Free, Dairy-Free, Grain-Free

2–3 Servings

I love making cobb salads at home, mainly because they break the "boring" salad stereotype (bacon and avocado make everything better). This balsamic dressing adds so much flavor and zing. The creamy factor comes from the avocado, which turns it from a vinaigrette to a wonderfully thick and velvety salad dressing.

2 eggs
1 teaspoon garlic powder
½ teaspoon paprika
½ teaspoon onion powder
½ teaspoon salt
¼ teaspoon black pepper
1 chicken breast
1 tablespoon extra-virgin olive oil
2 slices all-natural bacon
5–6 cups chopped romaine lettuce
1 tomato, sliced thin
1 avocado, sliced thin
1 whole carrot, grated

Creamy Balsamic Dressing:
½ cup balsamic vinegar
⅓ cup extra-virgin olive oil
½ avocado
1 garlic clove
¼ teaspoon salt
Dash of black pepper

1. Fill a small saucepan ¼ way with water and bring it to a boil. Place the eggs in the boiling water for 10–12 minutes for hard-boiled eggs.

2. For the chicken, in a small bowl mix together the garlic powder, paprika, onion powder, salt, and black pepper. Season the chicken breast well on both sides. Heat a skillet to medium heat with the olive oil, then cook your chicken breast about 10–12 minutes (flipping halfway through) until the chicken is cooked through and no longer pink. While the chicken is cooking, in the same skillet, add the two pieces of bacon and cook until the bacon is crisp.

3. Slice the cooked chicken breast into thin pieces. Peel the hard-boiled eggs and dice them, then crumble the cooked bacon.

4. For the creamy balsamic dressing, place all ingredients in a food processor and process until completely smooth.

5. In a large bowl, toss together the romaine lettuce, tomato, avocado, carrots, egg, chicken, and bacon. Serve with a side of the creamy balsamic dressing.

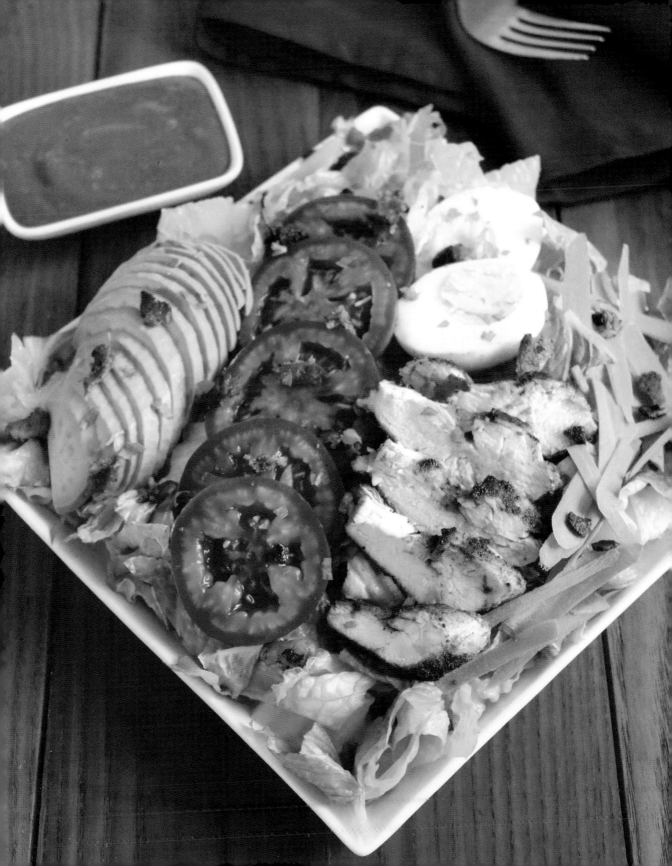

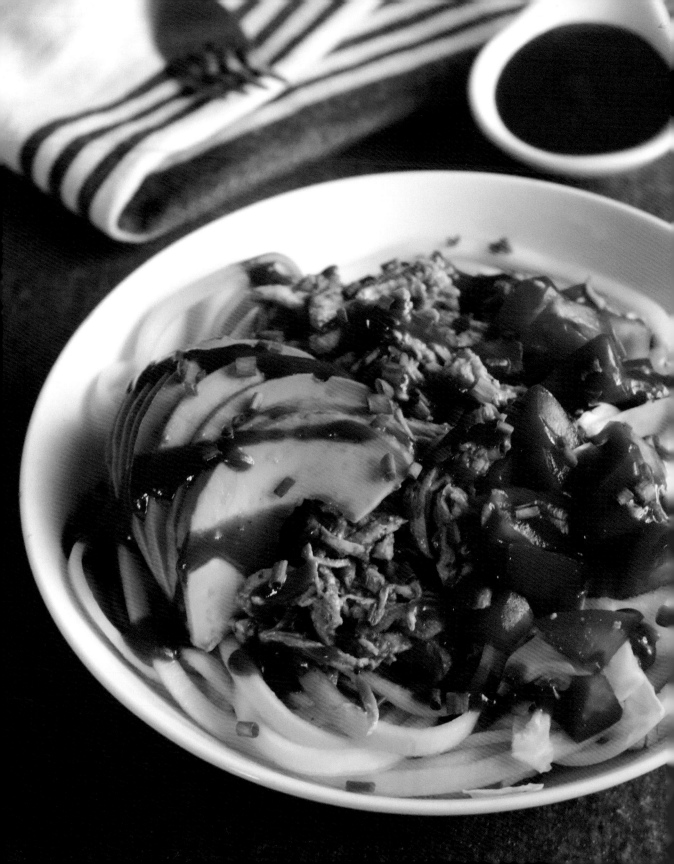

BBQ CHICKEN ZUCCHINI NOODLE BOWL

Gluten-Free, Dairy-Free, Grain-Free

Single Serving

Jason loves anything involving barbeque sauce, so I make this for lunch for him all the time because it's easy and totally satisfying. Zucchini noodles are light, yet filling, and a great replacement for pasta. They are simple to make using a vegetable spiralizer (something I highly recommend getting).

½ cup shredded cooked chicken
2 tablespoons barbeque sauce
1 medium sized zucchini, spiralized
¼ cup shredded cabbage
¼ cup diced tomatoes
½ avocado, sliced thin
1 teaspoon minced chives

> *TIP:* When using a store-bought barbeque sauce, I always try to find one that has all-natural ingredients and is sweetened with dates or honey instead of processed white sugar.

1. For this recipe, I usually poach a small chicken breast, then once it's cooked, I shred it. Mix the shredded chicken with 1 tablespoon of barbeque sauce and season with salt and pepper as desired.

2. For the zucchini noodles, you can either eat them raw or sauté them in a pan with 1 teaspoon of extra-virgin olive oil until they are softened, but not mushy.

3. Place the zucchini noodles in a bowl, then top with the barbeque chicken, cabbage, tomatoes, avocado, and chives, then drizzle in 1 tablespoon of barbeque sauce.

AVOCADO CHICKEN SALAD

Gluten-Free,
Dairy-Free, Grain-Free

1–2 Servings

This idea for the avocado chicken salad came to me because I absolutely love chicken salad, but Jason hates mayonnaise (more like he has a mayo-phobia). Even though you can make healthy homemade mayonnaise at home, you'll notice I don't have any mayonnaise recipes in this book. You can blame that one on Jason! The creaminess from the avocado is the perfect substitute for the mayo, and actually adds a wonderful flavor and buttery texture. I love the sweetness the raisins bring, and the celery gives it a nice crunch.

1 cup shredded cooked chicken
⅓ cup diced celery
2½ tablespoons unsweetened raisins
½ avocado, diced
1 tablespoon Dijon mustard
½ teaspoon salt
¼ teaspoon black pepper

Serve with cucumber and red bell pepper slices.

Place all ingredients in a bowl and mix together well. Serve the chicken salad with cucumber and red bell pepper slices for dipping.

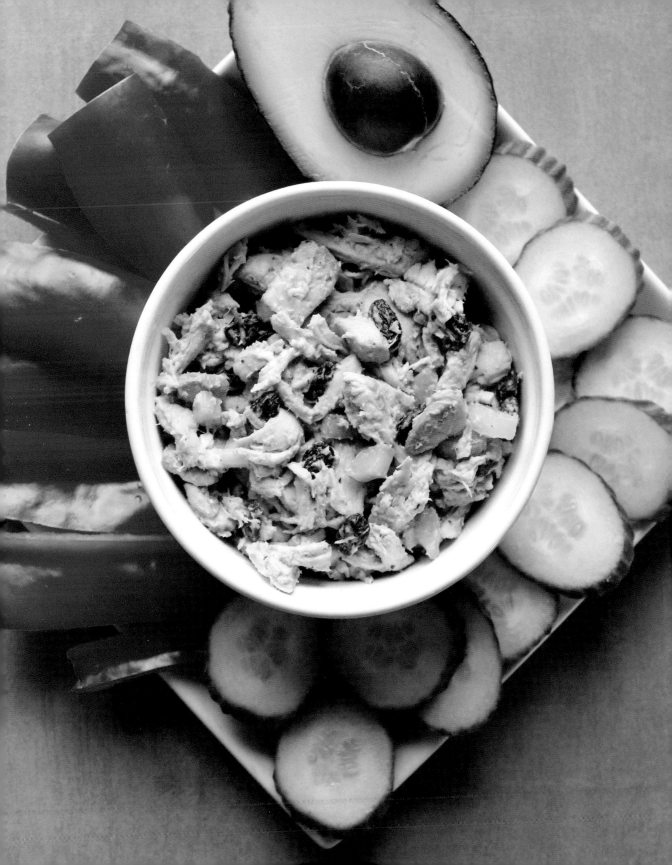

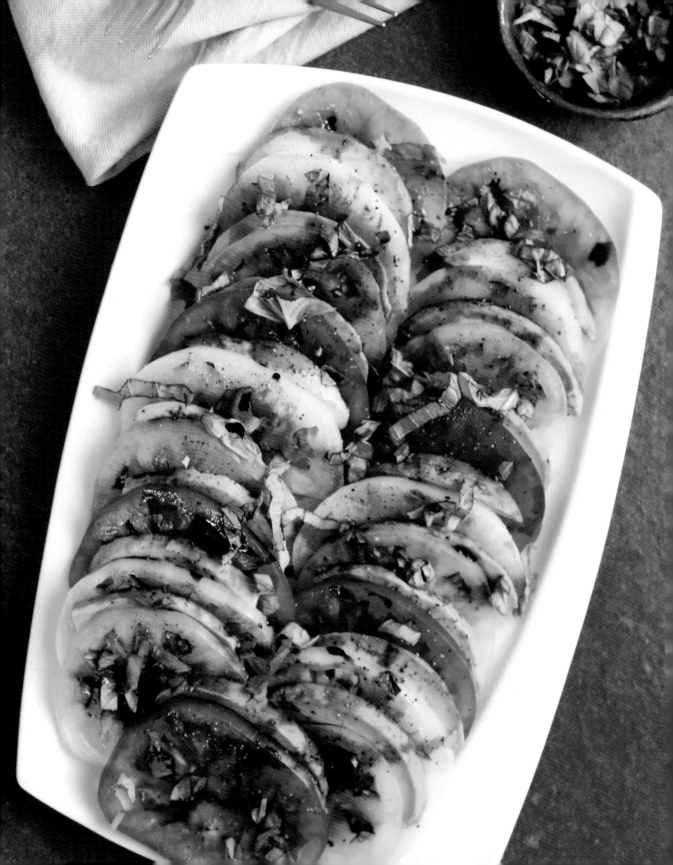

HEIRLOOM TOMATO AND AVOCADO SALAD WITH BASIL

Gluten-Free, Dairy-Free, Grain-Free, Vegan

2 Servings

One of my favorite things about our local farmer's market is they have a wonderful stand with fresh, organic heirloom tomatoes. Heirloom's come from seeds that have been handed down for generations (at least 50 years old) in a particular region, and hand-selected by farmers for a specific trait. That's where the variety of beautiful colors come from. This salad is so fresh and vibrant, and is balanced by the sweet acidity from the balsamic reduction.

1½–2 pounds heirloom tomatoes, sliced thin
2 medium avocados, sliced thin
¼ teaspoon salt
Black pepper, as desired
¼ cup fresh basil, roughly chopped

Balsamic Reduction:
⅓ cup balsamic vinegar

1. To make the balsamic reduction, pour the vinegar in a small saucepan and bring it to a rapid boil. Reduce the heat to low-medium and allow the sauce to simmer for 10–15 minutes or until the balsamic vinegar coats the back of the spoon. Remove from the heat and set aside.

2. To assemble the salad, stack the heirloom slices overlapping on one another on a long plate. Place avocado slices in between each tomato slice. Season the tomatoes with salt and pepper, then top with the fresh basil and drizzle the balsamic reduction all over.

NOTE: This salad is also nicely paired with a salty all-natural cured meat, such as a prosciutto.

TIP: Making a balsamic reduction can be tricky and it can turn into a black tar within seconds if you're not careful. Constantly check the reduction every 30 seconds or so to make sure it doesn't burn.

BAKED CHICKEN TAQUITOS WITH GUACAMOLE

Gluten-Free, Dairy-Free

Makes about 24 Taquitos

Growing up, I always loved taquitos, and they're something my mom made quite often, so I wanted to create a healthy rendition for Jason. These baked taquitos come out crispy on the outside and soft on the inside, and are really amazing. I like to make these for dinner or as an appetizer when friends come over—they get snatched up immediately every time!

Filling:

5 cups diced cooked chicken
½ cup canned green chili peppers
⅓ cup minced cilantro
1½ teaspoons salt
½ teaspoon paprika
½ teaspoon cumin
½ teaspoon garlic powder
2 tablespoons lime juice
24 corn tortillas
Coconut oil, for brushing

Guacamole:

3 medium avocados
⅓ cup minced cilantro
¼ cup minced red onions
½ cup diced tomatoes
1 tablespoon + 1 teaspoon lime juice
½ teaspoon salt
½ jalapeño, seeds removed and minced

1. Preheat your oven to 425 degrees.

2. In a bowl, mix together all filling ingredients (everything except tortillas and oil) and set aside. Put 5–6 tortillas at a time between a paper or kitchen towel and microwave for 15–20 seconds until the tortillas become soft and pliable for rolling.

3. Place a spoonful of the chicken filling towards the end of the corn tortilla (being careful not to overfill the taquito and making sure you leave space at the edges so the filling doesn't spill out) and roll the taquito as tightly as possible. With the seam side facing down, secure the taquito with a toothpick. Lightly grease a baking sheet and place the taquitos (seam side down) on the sheet, not touching one another. Brush the tops of the taquitos in coconut oil and bake for 15–20 minutes or until the ends are crispy.

4. For the guacamole, mix all ingredients together in a bowl. Serve the taquitos with the guacamole for dipping.

> **TIP:** If you aren't serving these as an appetizer for a party, you can place the extras in a ziplock bag and freeze for later use.

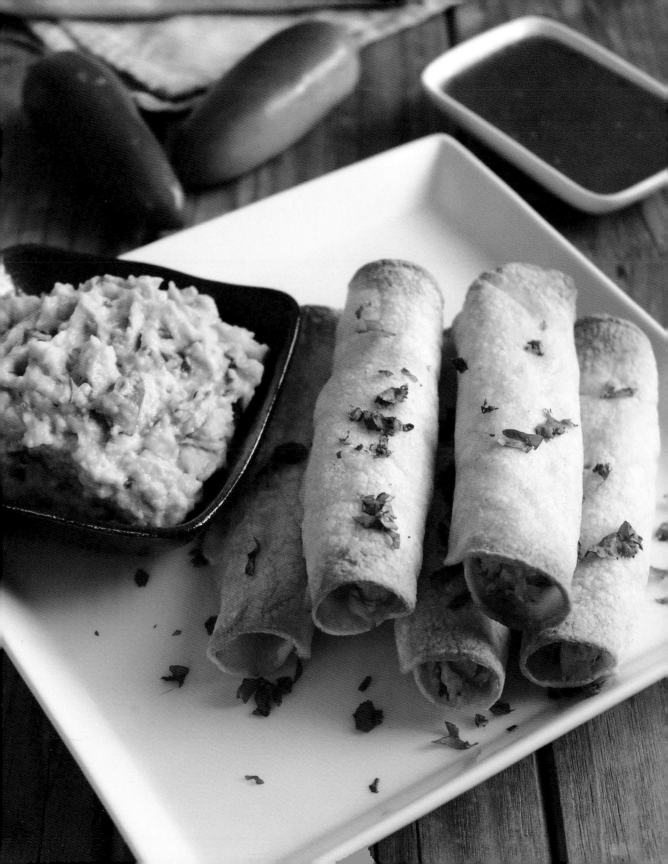

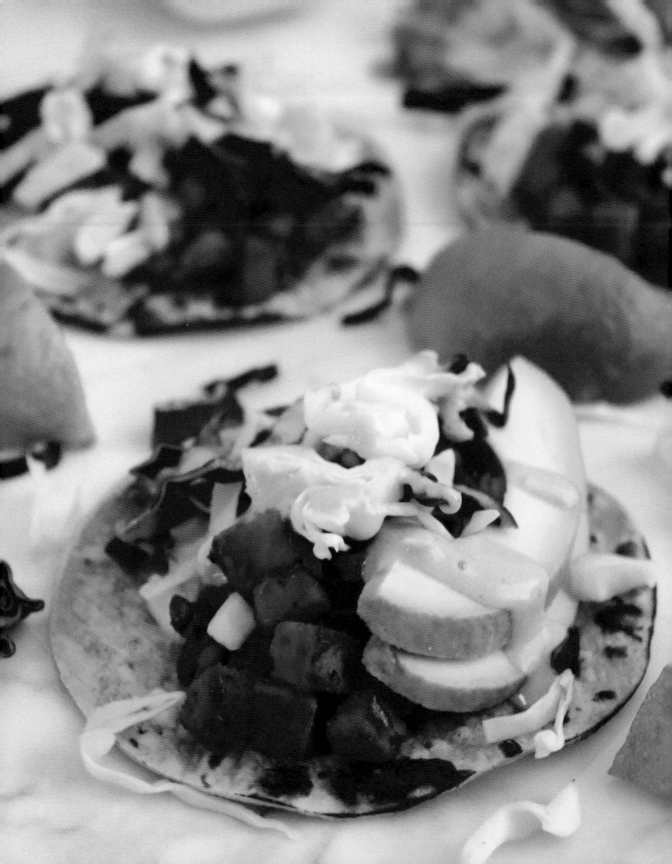

SWEET POTATO TACOS WITH SRIRACHA-TAHINI SAUCE

Gluten-Free, Dairy-Free, Vegan

Makes About 12 Tacos

These are my "Meatless Monday" go-to tacos. The filling is surprisingly meaty from the mushrooms, and you won't believe the sriracha-tahini sauce is dairy-free! These little tacos are finger-licking good.

Filling:
3 cups diced sweet potatoes
1 cup minced red onions
2 tablespoons coconut oil
2 cups chopped white mushrooms
½ teaspoon salt
¼ teaspoon black pepper
½ teaspoon paprika
½ teaspoon garlic powder
¼ teaspoon chili powder

Sriracha-Tahini Sauce:
⅓ cup tahini paste
½ cup coconut milk
1 tablespoon sriracha
   (recipe on page 128)
1 tablespoon lime juice
2 teaspoons honey
1 garlic clove

10–12 mini corn tortillas
1 large avocado, sliced thin
1 cup shredded cabbage
Fresh minced cilantro, as desired

Serve with lime wedges

1. For the taco filling, place the sweet potatoes in a small pot of boiling water. Par-boil them for about 3–4 minutes until they have softened, but not turned into mush. Drain the sweet potatoes and set them aside. In a skillet, sauté the onions in 1 tablespoon of coconut oil until translucent. Add in the mushrooms and continue to sauté on high heat until the moisture from the mushrooms has absorbed. Add in the sweet potatoes, 1 tablespoon of coconut oil and all seasonings. Sauté the filling until the sweet potatoes are browned and crisp (8–10 minutes).

2. For the sriracha-tahini sauce, place all ingredients in a food processor and process until the sauce is completely smooth. Transfer to a small bowl.

3. Heat the corn tortillas on a burner about 10–15 seconds per side. To assemble the tacos, spoon the filling on each corn tortilla then top with sliced avocado, cabbage, cilantro, and the sriracha-tahini sauce. Squeeze fresh lime juice over each taco.

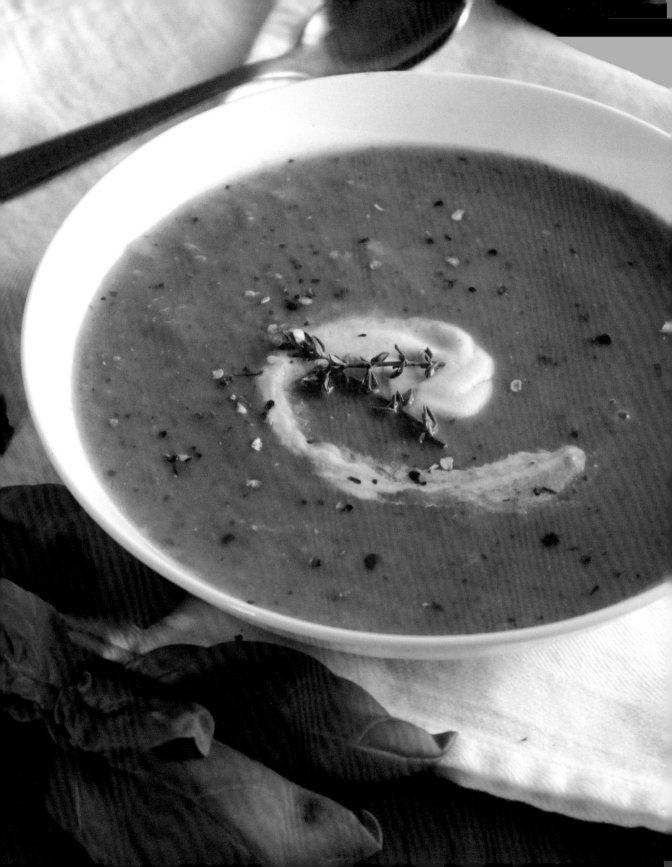

Soups

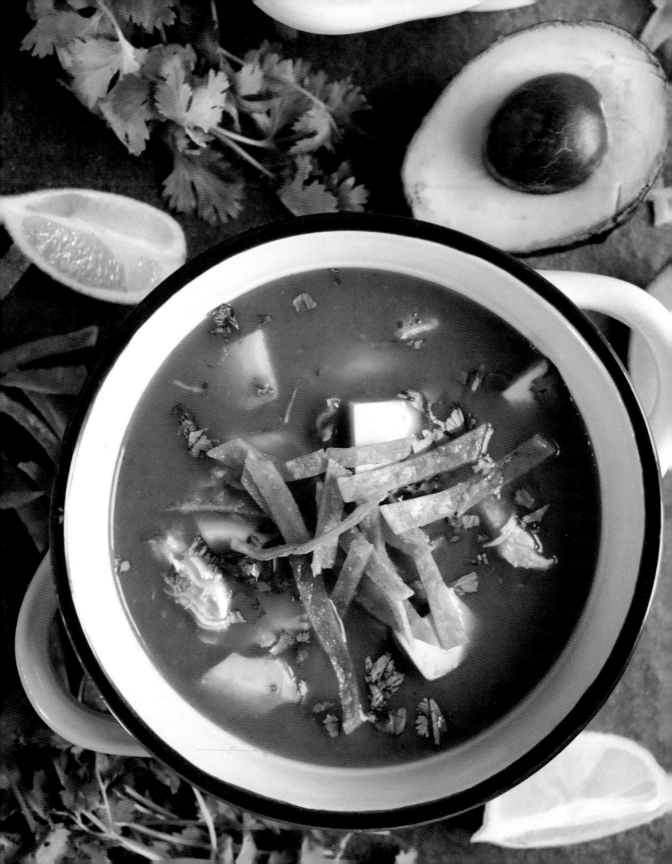

CHICKEN TORTILLA SOUP

Gluten-Free, Dairy-Free

3–4 Servings

This soup is packed with so much flavor, texture, and complexity. The broth is silky smooth with rich, smoky flavors, and I love the creaminess the avocado adds, then you get that wonderful crunch from the tortilla strips. Jason requests this soup all the time, and once you try making this recipe you'll understand why!

1 cup chopped white onions
5 garlic cloves
1 jalapeño, sliced in half
2 tablespoons extra-virgin olive oil
14.5 ounces canned, diced
    tomatoes
4 cups low-sodium chicken broth
1 teaspoon cumin
½ teaspoon chili powder
½ teaspoon paprika
1½ teaspoons salt
2 cups cooked shredded chicken

Toppings:
1 cup corn tortilla strips
    (See to the right for directions)
2 tablespoons coconut oil
Dash of salt
Avocado, diced
    (about ⅓ cup per person)
Fresh minced cilantro, as desired

Serve with lime wedges

1. In a Dutch oven or stockpot, sauté the onions, garlic cloves, and jalapeño in olive oil for about 5 minutes or until the onions are translucent. Don't worry about cutting anything small, as you will puree the soup. Add the diced tomatoes, and cooked onions, garlic, and jalapeño to a blender and blend until everything is completely smooth. Add the tomato puree back into your pot along with the chicken broth. Add in the cumin, chili powder, paprika, and salt. Bring the broth to a boil then reduce the heat to low and let the broth simmer, covered for 20–30 minutes.

2. For the tortilla strips, simply take a corn tortilla and use scissors to cut the tortilla into long, thin strips. Heat the coconut oil in a skillet and on medium-high heat, fry the tortilla strips until they are crispy. Transfer the strips to a paper towel to catch any oil, then sprinkle them with salt.

3. Once the broth is done simmering, add in the cooked chicken to the broth. Spoon the soup into individual bowls and top with the diced avocado, cilantro, tortilla strips, and squeeze lime juice over the top.

HOMEMADE CHICKEN BROTH

Gluten-Free, Dairy-Free, Grain-Free

Yields 14–15 Cups

There is nothing quite like homemade chicken broth. Once you make chicken broth at home, it's really hard to go back to using store-bought broth because the flavor doesn't even compare to the rich, buttery flavor of chicken broth when it's homemade. This recipe is incredibly easy and what I love is you can use the meat from the chicken carcass for soup or other quick and easy meals throughout the week.

1 (4–4.5 pound) whole chicken
2 celery stalks, cut in halves
2 whole carrots, cut in halves
1 head of garlic, top cut off
1 bunch of parsley
1 large yellow onion, cut in fourths
2 rosemary sprigs
5 thyme sprigs
3 bay leaves
1 tablespoon white peppercorn
1 teaspoon coriander
4 quarts water
2 teaspoons salt

1. Place all ingredients (except the salt) in a large stockpot, adding in the water last. Bring the water to a boil, then reduce the heat to low and let the broth sit uncovered for 2–3 hours, stirring the ingredients every so often.

2. Place a strainer or colander over another large pot. Pour the simmering chicken broth into the strainer so that the strainer catches the chicken carcass and all other ingredients and the stockpot below holds the strained broth. Once the chicken carcass cools, you can shred the chicken meat and use it immediately or save for later use. Dispose of the simmered vegetables.

3. Add the salt to the strained chicken broth and once it cools, pour the broth into mason jars or airtight sealed containers and place it in the refrigerator overnight before use. When you go to use the chicken broth after it has been refrigerated, the fat will separate and turn gelatinous. This is completely normal! Once you re-heat the broth, the fat will melt back into a liquid and it adds so much body and flavor.

> *FACT:* Chicken broth is so healing for our bodies—especially when you make it homemade and are getting all the nutrients from the bones that have minerals, collagen, and gelatin. You can actually save the chicken bones from this recipe and turn them into a bone broth by simmering them for 12–24 hours.

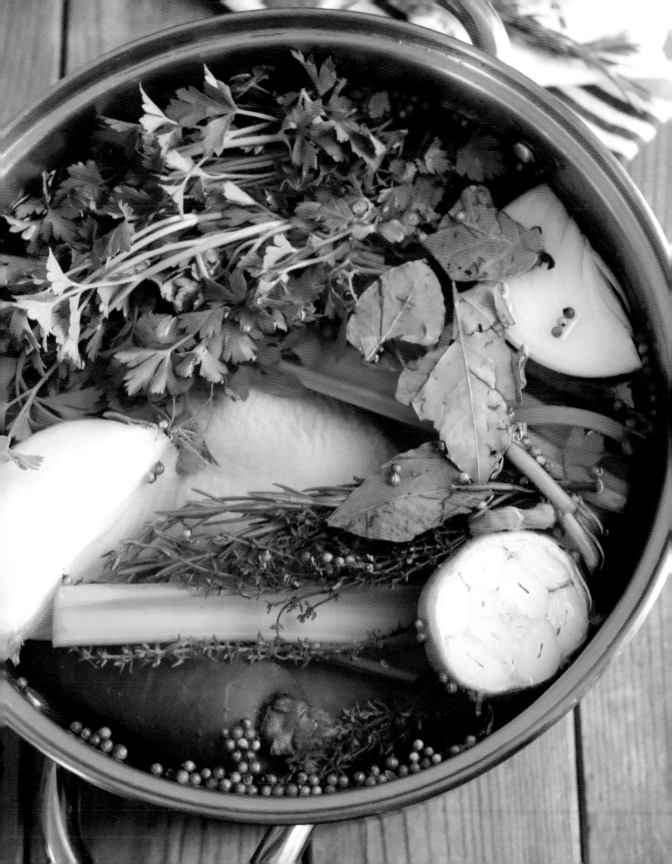

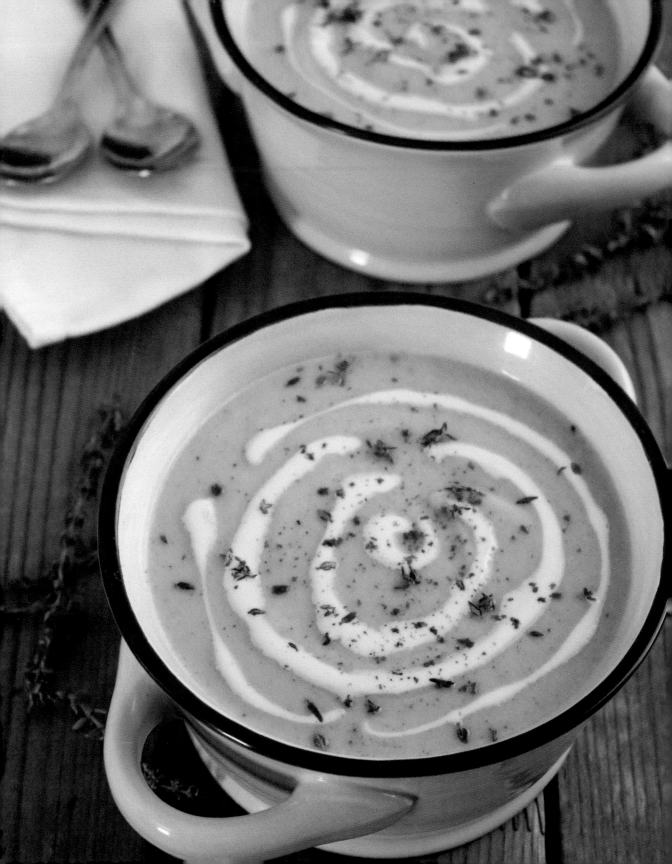

BUTTERNUT SQUASH BISQUE

Gluten-Free, Dairy-Free, Grain-Free

Yields about 7 Cups (4 Servings)

Sometimes it's hard getting Jason to eat all of his vegetables, so I love to make him this soup because it is pureed so I can sneak a lot of vegetables in there without him knowing! This soup is velvety smooth, and so aromatic from the nutmeg and thyme; it makes you feel warmed from the inside out.

4 cups cubed butternut squash
2 celery stalks, chopped
2 large carrots, chopped
2 cups yellow onions, chopped
4 whole garlic cloves
2 teaspoons minced thyme
2 tablespoons extra-virgin olive oil
1 cup coconut cream
   (See note below)
2 cups low-sodium chicken broth
½ teaspoon nutmeg
¼ teaspoon cinnamon
¼ teaspoon cayenne pepper
1½ teaspoons salt

Toppings:

Additional coconut cream for drizzling
Fresh thyme, as desired
Dash of cayenne pepper
   (For added spice)

1. Fill a medium-sized stockpot with water and bring it to a boil. Add in the butternut squash, celery, and carrots. Boil for 8–10 minutes or until everything is softened and fork tender. Drain and set aside.

2. In a Dutch oven or large stockpot, sauté the onions, whole garlic cloves, and thyme in olive oil about 5 minutes or until the onions are translucent. You don't need to chop anything too small as you will puree it afterwards. Add the boiled butternut squash, carrots, celery, onions, garlic, and thyme to a high-power blender along with the coconut cream and chicken broth and blend everything on high speed until the soup is completely smooth. Transfer the pureed soup back to the pot. If you have an immersion blender you can skip this step and simply place everything in your Dutch oven and blend until the soup is smooth. Add in all the spices and allow to soup to simmer on low at least 30 minutes before serving.

3. Top the soup with additional coconut cream, thyme, and cayenne pepper.

NOTE: I love to add crispy mushrooms to the top of this soup! Sauté thinly sliced mushrooms in olive oil until they are browned and crispy (about 10 minutes) and sprinkle the mushrooms with salt.

TIP: For the coconut cream, place a can of full-fat coconut milk in the refrigerator for at least 12 hours. Remove the can from the refrigerator (being careful not to shake the can), open the can and scoop out the cream that forms at the top.

KALE AND GNOCCHI SOUP WITH CHICKEN SAUSAGE

Gluten-Free, Dairy-Free

4–5 Servings

I like to think of gnocchi as little fluffy pillows of heaven. Gnocchi are thick, soft potato dumplings and they go wonderfully in this soup. The kale adds a hearty texture and the Italian chicken sausage brings along a great kick from the spice. I highly recommend making this recipe using my homemade chicken broth from page 88 for a richer, deeper flavor.

½ pound spicy Italian chicken sausage
2 tablespoons extra-virgin olive oil
5 garlic cloves, minced
7 cups low-sodium chicken broth
1 cup coconut milk
3 cups roughly chopped packed kale
⅓ cup roughly chopped basil
1 teaspoon salt
½ teaspoon black pepper
9 ounces pre-made gluten-free gnocchi

1. If your chicken sausage is not already ground, then cut the casing off and squeeze it out. In a Dutch oven or large stockpot, sauté the chicken sausage in olive oil, breaking the sausage apart as it cooks down. Once the sausage is nearly cooked, add in the garlic and sauté it for another minute or so. Now add in all ingredients except the gnocchi. Bring the soup to a boil, then reduce the heat to low and allow it to simmer 30–60 minutes.

2. Before serving the soup, add in the gnocchi. Gnocchi cooks fast, typically within 30 seconds, and the gnocchi will float at the top of the soup once they are ready. Serve immediately.

NOTE: The brand I use of pre-made gluten-free gnocchi is Delallo. It's actually made in Italy and has all-natural ingredients. A lot of brands of gnocchi are made with wheat flour so be sure to always check your ingredients labels.

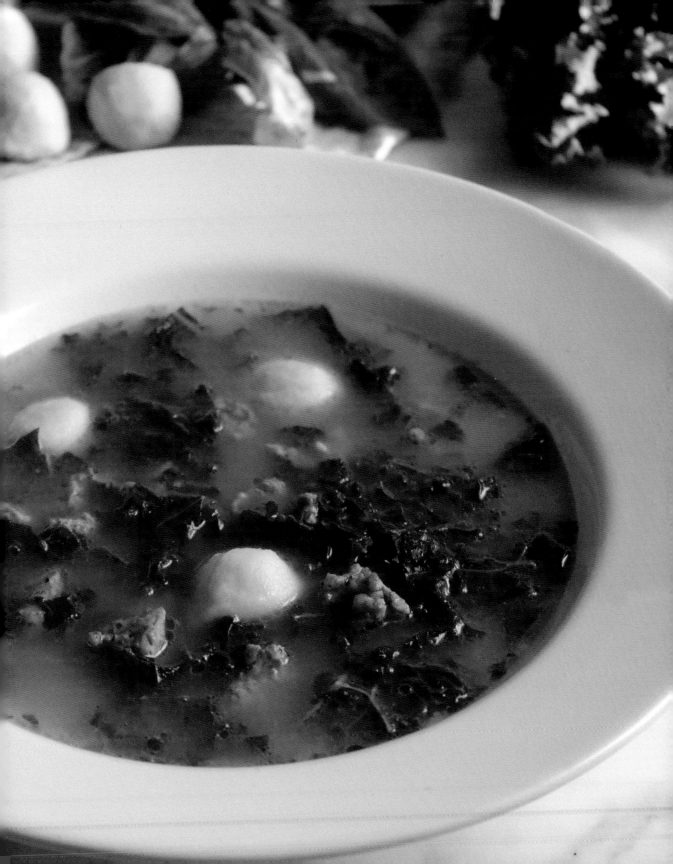

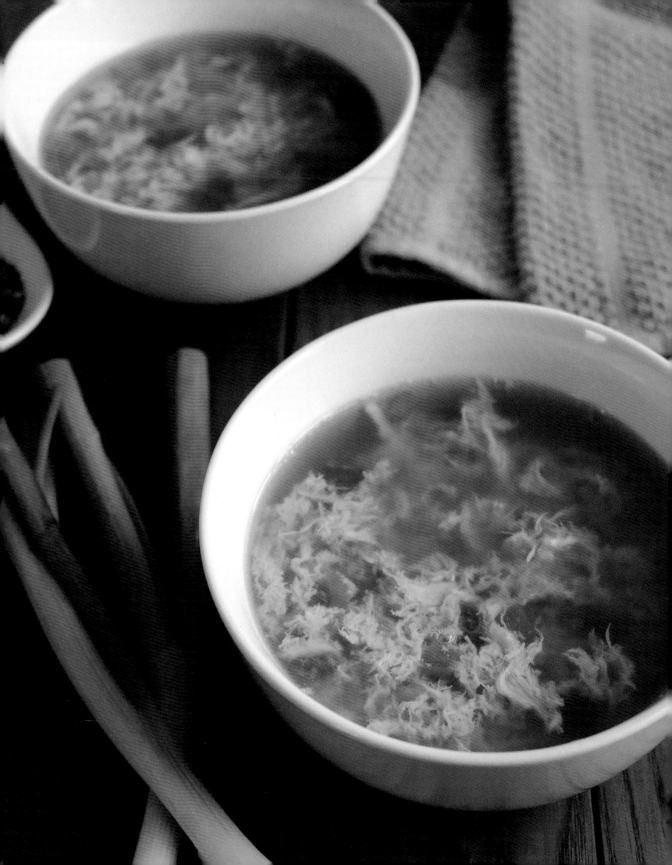

EGG DROP SOUP

Gluten-Free, Dairy-Free, Grain-Free

Makes 3–4 Servings

Egg drop soup is a traditional Chinese soup made of wispy, beaten eggs in a broth. This soup is super simple, has minimal ingredients, and you can add any vegetable or protein as you see fit. I love watching the silky eggs cook almost immediately as your pour them into the boiling broth—it's strangely mesmerizing!

6 cups low-sodium chicken broth
2 tablespoons coconut aminos
2 inches ginger, sliced into 4 rounds
1 teaspoon sesame oil
½ teaspoon garlic powder
1 cup chopped green onions
¼ teaspoon crushed red pepper
½ teaspoon salt
4 eggs

1. In a Dutch oven or stockpot, add in all ingredients, except the eggs. Bring the soup to a boil, then reduce the heat and let it simmer on low for 20–30 minutes. Remove the ginger pieces and discard.

2. In a small bowl, whisk together the eggs. Bring the soup to a rapid boil and pour the eggs into the soup while whisking the soup constantly as you pour the eggs in. The eggs will cook immediately and become wispy and silky smooth. If you don't whisk the soup fast in a constant motion while pouring the eggs in, you will end up with scrambled eggs so this step is important. Serve the soup immediately.

> **NOTE:** Most egg drop soup recipes call for cornstarch, but I find it completely unnecessary and the whisked eggs give the soup great body without using the cornstarch method.

TOM KHA GAI (THAI COCONUT SOUP)

Gluten-Free, Dairy-Free, Grain-Free

4–6 Servings

Tom Kha Gai is a spicy and sour coconut soup. It's one of our absolute favorite soups that we always order at Thai restaurants. The flavor is so unique and comes from the fresh lemongrass stalks and Thai chilies. If you love Thai food, then you will love this recipe! The cooking process is simple and you end up with the most aromatic, savory soup.

6 cups low-sodium chicken broth

2 cups full-fat coconut milk

4 cups roughly chopped white mushrooms

2 lemongrass stalks, cut into 2-inch pieces, then smashed

2 inches ginger, sliced into 4 rounds

2 Thai chilies (If you can't find these, you can use 1 red jalapeño, sliced in half)

1 cup diced green onions

2 tablespoons lime juice

1 teaspoon salt

3 tablespoons coconut aminos

1 tablespoon honey

2 cups shredded cooked chicken

Serve the soup topped with fresh cilantro and lime wedges

1. Place all ingredients (except the chicken) in a Dutch oven or stockpot. Bring the soup to a boil, then let it simmer on low, covered for 45–60 minutes. This will really bring out the flavors of the lemongrass and ginger. Once the soup is done simmering, remove the lemongrass and ginger pieces with a slotted spoon and discard.

2. Add the cooked chicken into the soup then serve the soup topped with fresh cilantro and lime juice.

> **TIP:** If you haven't cooked with lemongrass before, it can be a bit tricky. When you cut the stalks then smash each piece, it will release the flavors from the inside of the stalk that is surrounded by the outer layers.

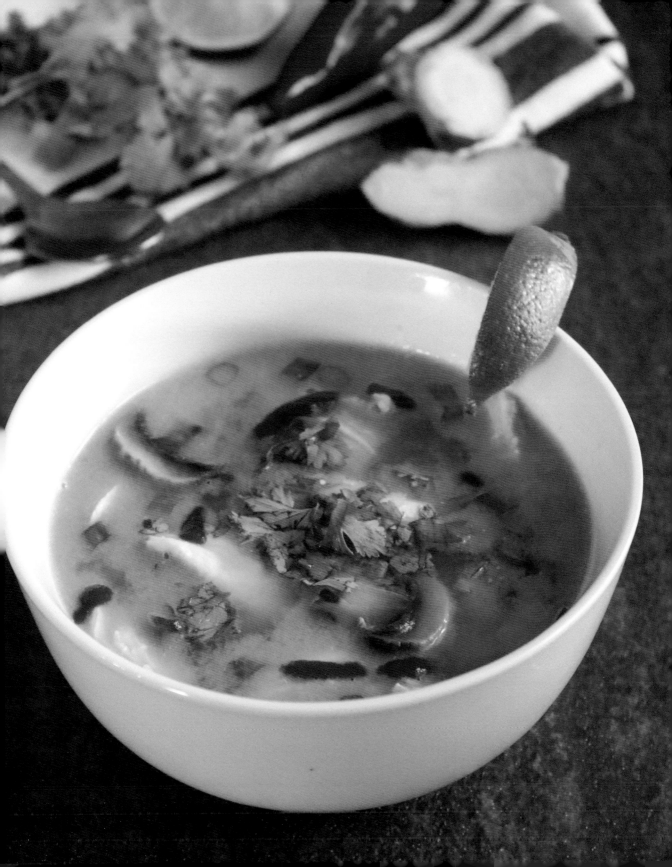

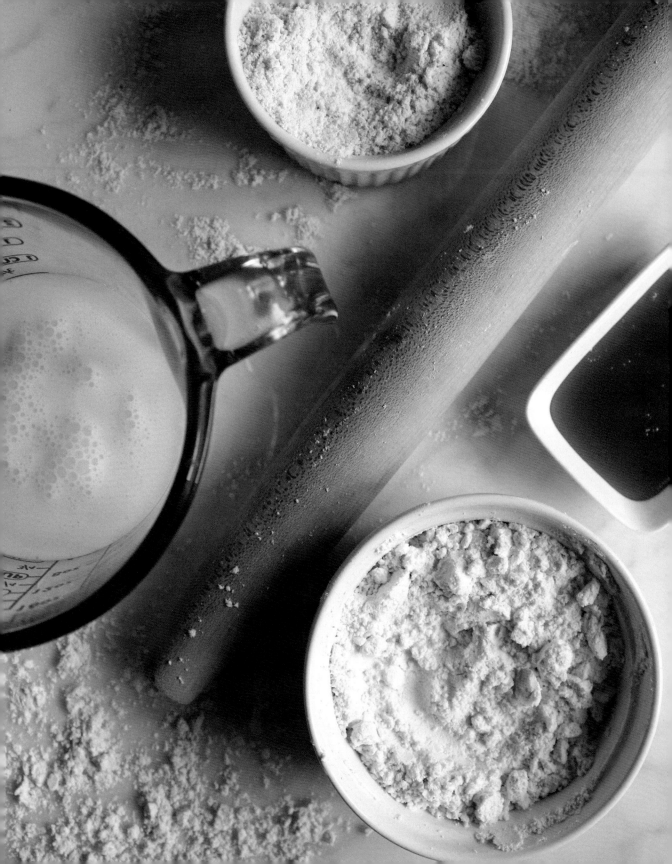

Breads

Once you go gluten-free, the first bummer is realizing that gluten-free bread is not and will never be the same as normal bread. You are never going to find a perfect gluten-free bread so it's a realization that if you do choose to eat gluten-free bread, the texture is going to be different. Gluten in bread is what causes the dough to swell and become elastic. It is a protein that forms when wheat flour and water mix together, and the gluten gives structure to the dough. If you have ever tried making gluten-free bread at home, you know it is sticky, hard to form, and a bit frustrating, to be honest.

However, that does not mean gluten-free bread isn't just as delicious! In fact, we are so used to the way things taste since going gluten-free a few years ago, we've actually come to prefer it. I love how crispy gluten-free pizza crusts get, and homemade gluten-free bread is so chewy and doughy, it's delightful.

For my bread recipes, I've listed the brand names of the gluten-free all-purpose flours that work best for that particular recipe. If you are going to make the recipe, I highly recommend using the brand listed or the outcome may be completely different. You can make a gluten-free all-purpose flour at home, but in order for gluten-free flour to work it has to combine a lot of different types of flours to get a good result and that can become tedious, not to mention expensive. The brands I've listed can easily be bought at your local grocery store or online.

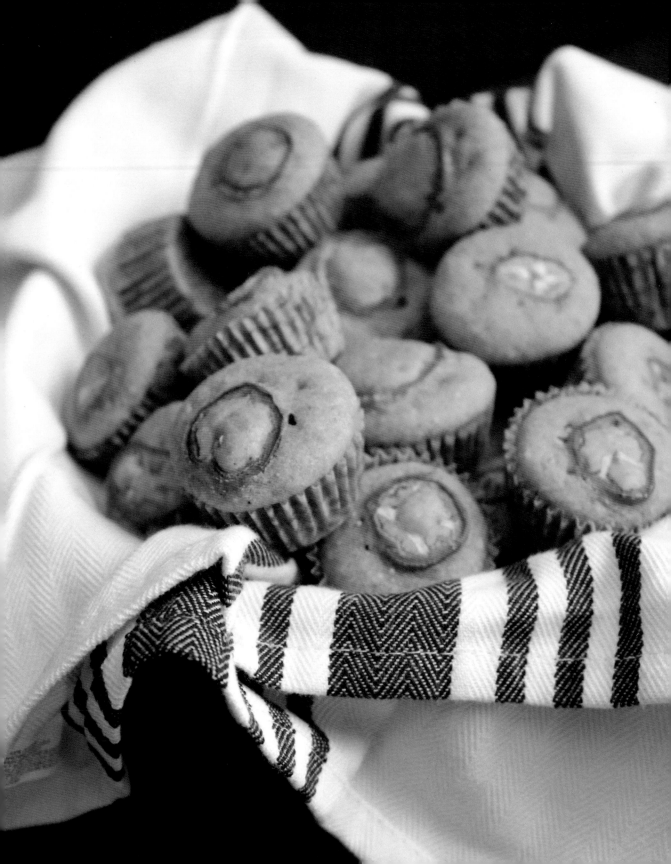

MINI JALAPEÑO-HONEY CORNBREAD MUFFINS

Gluten-Free, Dairy-Free, Vegetarian

Makes about 30 Mini Muffins

Every year, Jason and I go to a chili cook-off at one of our favorite local restaurants. It's tradition for Jason to make his famous spicy chili, and I make my mini-jalapeño cornbread muffins to go along with the chili. These are perfect little bite-sized muffins, and the sweet honey balances out the spicy peppers beautifully. These also get eaten up quick so I recommend making the whole batch!

30 mini muffin paper liners
1 cup yellow cornmeal (Arrowhead
    Mills Organic Yellow Cornmeal)
1 cup gluten-free all-purpose flour
    (Bob's Red Mill Gluten-Free
    All-Purpose Baking Flour)
½ teaspoon baking soda
½ teaspoon salt
1 cup full-fat coconut milk
⅓ cup honey
3 tablespoons unsweetened
    applesauce
1 egg
2 tablespoons extra-virgin olive oil
1–2 tablespoons minced jalapeños,
    seeds removed (depending on
    how spicy you want them)
30 thin slices of jalapeños (to top
    the muffins with)

1. Preheat your oven to 325 degrees.

2. Using a mini muffin baking pan, place a baking liner into each muffin slot.

3. In a large bowl, mix together the cornmeal, flour, baking soda, and salt. In a separate bowl, mix together the coconut milk, honey, applesauce, egg, olive oil, and minced jalapeño. Combine the wet ingredients in with the dry ingredients and make sure the batter is mixed well.

4. Scoop 1 tablespoon at a time of the batter into each baking cup. Place a thinly-sliced jalapeño on top of each muffin. Bake the muffins for 11–12 minutes. Remove the muffins from the oven and allow them to cool for 5 minutes. Serve warm.

ROSEMARY BREAD

Gluten-Free, Dairy-Free, Vegetarian

Makes One Loaf

This bread is absolutely amazing. The fresh rosemary gives it this earthiness, and if you use the flour listed below, the loaf comes out so soft and chewy. I like to serve this bread at dinner with a side of olive oil and balsamic to dip it in, at breakfast with jam, or you can even make a sandwich out of it! It's incredibly versatile.

1½ cups warm water

1 packet active dry yeast (¼ ounce)

2 tablespoons honey

3½ cups gluten-free all-purpose flour + more for kneading (Namaste Organic Perfect Gluten-Free Flour Blend)

1 tablespoon minced fresh rosemary

2 eggs

2 tablespoons extra-virgin olive oil

1 tablespoon apple cider vinegar

1½ teaspoons salt

NOTE: You can keep the bread in a sealed container in the refrigerator up to one week. When you use the bread, you need to put it in the toaster for a few minutes before serving. I always like to slightly undercook gluten-free bread as it can turn hard rather quickly.

1. In a bowl, combine the warm water, yeast, and honey, and let it sit about 10 minutes or until the yeast is activated and frothy. In another large bowl, combine the flour and rosemary. In a third bowl, combine the eggs, oil, apple cider vinegar, and salt. Now, combine all ingredients into the large bowl with the flour and mix everything together well.

2. Flour a dry, flat surface, and spoon the dough onto the floured surface. Flour the top of the dough and your hands, and gently knead the dough for 1–2 minutes. You may need to sprinkle more flour on top of the dough while you're kneading it if it becomes too sticky.

3. Grease a baking sheet and place the dough on the sheet. Form the dough into a bread loaf shape then cover the dough with a towel and let it sit in a warm place for 60 minutes while it rises.

4. Preheat your oven to 350 degrees. Bake the bread for 45–50 minutes. Remove the bread from the oven and allow it to cool for 10 minutes. Once the bread has cooled, slice it and serve warm.

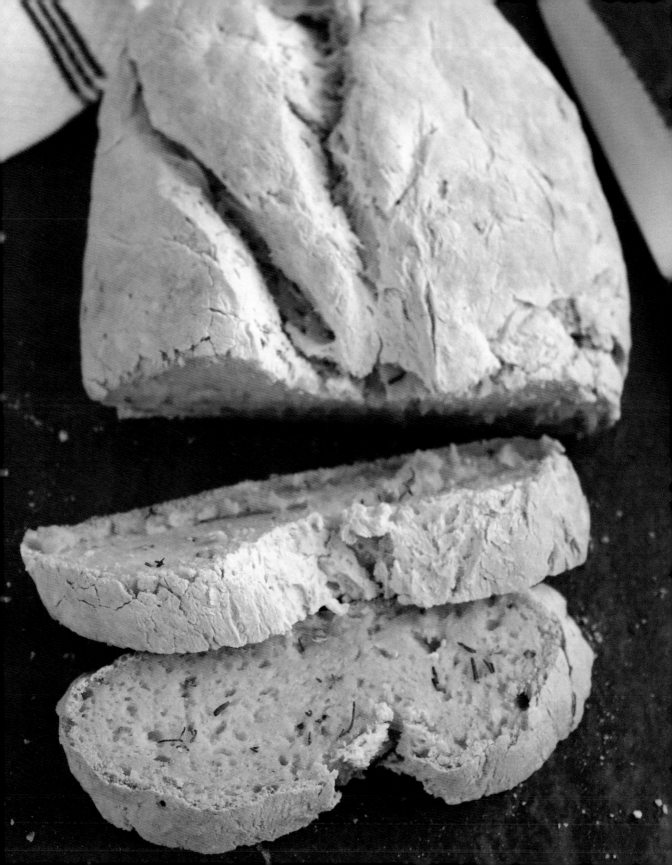

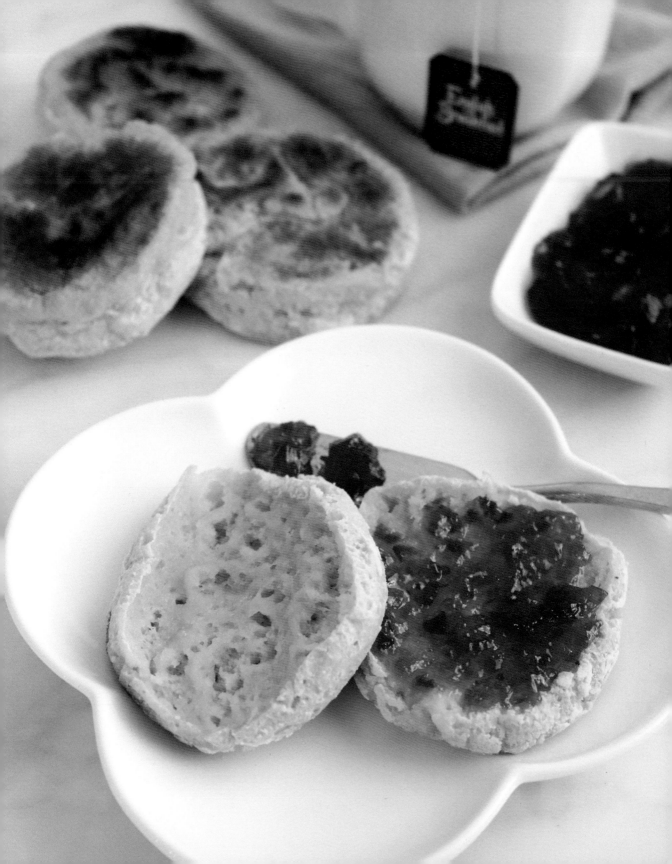

CRUMPETS

Gluten-Free, Dairy-Free, Vegetarian

Yields about 10 Crumpets

Crumpets are griddle cakes made from flour and yeast, and usually served with some type of jam. Growing up, we always had crumpets around the house, and they bring back such fond memories. Jason loves these warmed for breakfast with a cup of coffee or tea. They are crispy on the outside, and soft and chewy on the inside—and nothing short of spectacular.

2 cups all-purpose gluten-free flour + more for dusting (Namaste Organic Perfect Gluten-Free Flour Blend)
1 packet active dry yeast (¼ ounce)
1 teaspoon salt
1½ cups almond milk
1 tablespoon honey
1 tablespoon extra-virgin olive oil

1. In a large bowl, combine the flour, yeast, and salt.

2. In a small saucepan, add in the almond milk, honey, and olive oil. Stir the mixture on medium-low heat about two minutes until it is hot (not boiling).

3. Pour the hot mixture into the flour bowl and combine all ingredients well, forming into a dough. Dust a dry, flat surface with flour, and spoon the dough onto the surface. Flour the top of the dough and your hands, and knead for 1–2 minutes. You may need to sprinkle more flour on top of the dough if it becomes too sticky to knead. Form the dough into a large ball, cover it with a towel, and let it sit for one hour to rest and rise.

4. Flour your hands again and flatten out the dough to be ¼–½ inch in thickness. Using a circular 3-inch-wide cookie cutter, cut the dough into 10 equal pieces. When you've cut the crumpet pieces out, form the pieces of dough that are left over into another ball and repeat the steps until the dough is all used up.

5. Grease a skillet on medium heat with a non-stick cooking spray. Place each crumpet on the skillet (the dough is very delicate, so be gentle) and let it cook for 8 minutes on the first side, then flip them over and continue to cook them for 2–4 more minutes. It's best to undercook the dough so they end up soft on the inside.

6. You can serve the crumpets immediately, topped with jam, peanut butter, or honey, or you can store them in a sealed container up to one week. Once they have been refrigerated, the crumpets are best sliced in half then toasted.

BANANA BREAD

Gluten-Free, Dairy-Free, Vegetarian

Makes One Loaf

To me there is no better smell than the aroma of homemade banana bread baking in the oven. It's delicious served warm with a cup of coffee in the morning, as a dessert with a scoop of coconut ice cream, or for anytime of the day, really. This banana bread recipe comes out so moist, soft, and flavorful. I could eat this whole loaf easily by myself; it's that scrumptious!

1½ cups gluten-free all-purpose flour (Bob's Red Mill Gluten-Free All-Purpose Baking Flour)
1 teaspoon baking soda
½ teaspoon nutmeg
1 teaspoon cinnamon
½ teaspoon salt
4 large ripe bananas, mashed
2 eggs
2 tablespoons almond milk
½ cup coconut oil
½ cup honey

1. Pre-heat your oven to 325 degrees.

2. In a large bowl mix together the flour, baking soda, nutmeg, cinnamon, and salt. In a separate bowl, mix together the mashed bananas, eggs, almond milk, coconut oil, and honey. Combine the wet ingredients in with the dry ingredients, and using an electric hand mixer, combine the batter until no clumps are formed.

3. Grease a 5x9-inch loaf pan with a non-stick cooking spray. Pour the batter into the greased bread pan. Bake the banana bread uncovered for 60 minutes. Once it's done cooking, remove the banana bread from the oven and allow it to cool for 10–15 minutes. Gently remove the banana bread from the pan, then slice it and serve warm.

> **TIP:** The riper the bananas, the better! You want the peel as brown as possible. This is what really moistens the bread and gives it the best flavor.

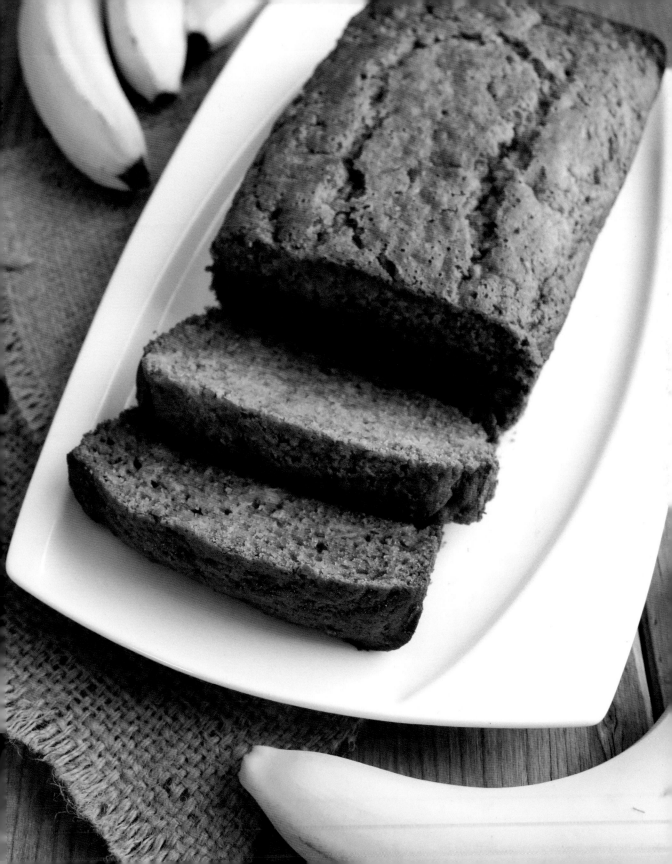

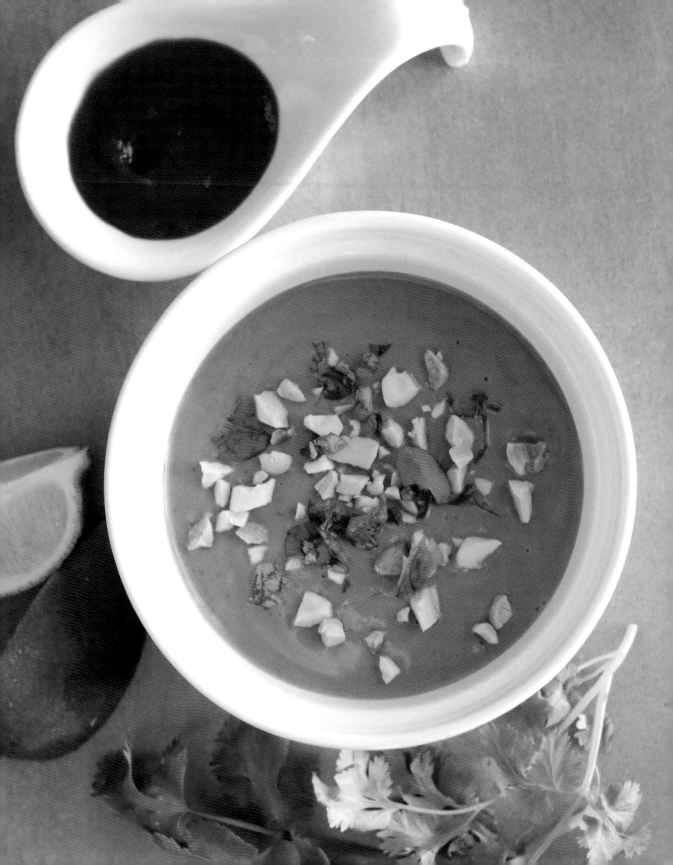

Nut Cheeses, Milks, Sauces, and Dips

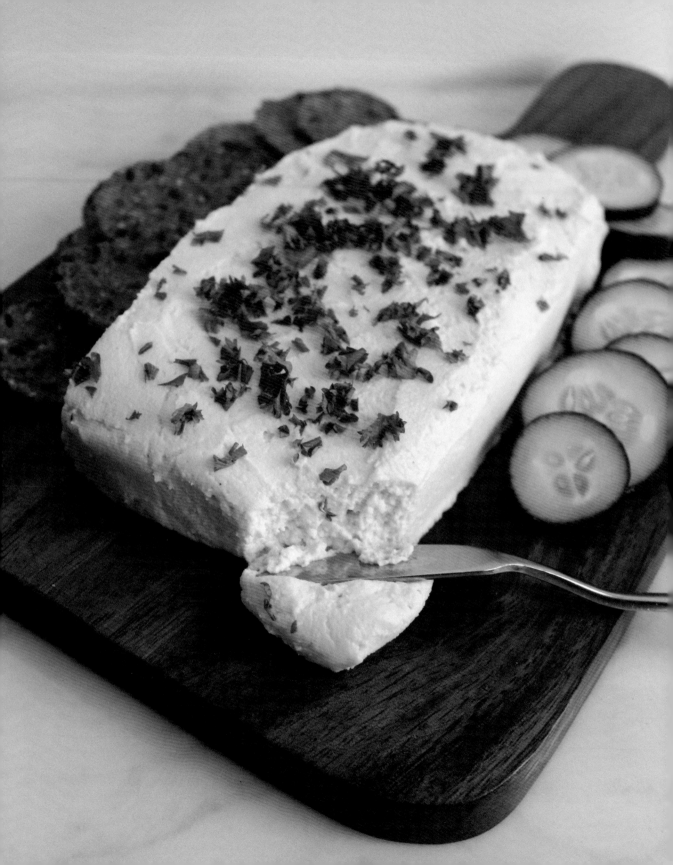

MACADAMIA CREAM CHEESE

Gluten-Free, Dairy-Free, Grain-Free, Vegan

Yields 2 Cups

This raw macadamia cream cheese tastes so much like conventional dairy cream cheese it's incredible! The process of making it does take some time and patience, but I promise you it's well worth the wait. It's wonderful spread over my Sweet Potato Toast (page 28), used to dip veggies and rice crackers in, or you can use it in place of any of your favorite cream cheese recipes—the texture is nearly identical!

2 cups raw, unsalted macadamia nuts
1½ cups filtered water
2 teaspoons lemon juice
1½ teaspoons salt

*You will need a fine mesh cheesecloth

1. In a high-power blender, blend the macadamia nuts, water, lemon juice, and salt, until completely smooth.

2. First, lay a plate down on a flat surface, and place a colander on top of the plate. Line the colander with the cheesecloth. Pour the macadamia mixture onto the cheesecloth. At this point the macadamia cheese will be mush—don't worry, that's normal! Twist the top of the cheesecloth and secure it with a clip, making sure none of the macadamia mixture is visible.

3. Next, place a smaller plate that fits inside the colander on top of the cheesecloth. You want to put a weighted object on top of that plate because the weight will force all of the moisture out of the macadamia nuts, forcing it through the cheesecloth, then the liquid will fall onto the bottom plate. I like to use my 84-ounce jar of coconut oil as the object to weigh the cream cheese down.

4. Leave your macadamia cream cheese set-up in a warm, dry place for at least 16 hours and up to 24 hours. No need to touch it! Through this time, you will see the liquid slowly coming out of the cheesecloth, through the colander, and fall onto the plate.

5. Remove the cream cheese from the cloth. The cream cheese should be firm, yet soft and completely moldable. I like to put the cream cheese in aluminum foil and mold it into a rectangular shape, then cover it with the foil and place it in an air-tight sealed container.

6. Store the macadamia cream cheese in the refrigerator for up to one week.

LEMON-HERB CASHEW RICOTTA

Gluten-Free, Dairy-Free, Grain-Free, Vegan
Yields about 3 Cups

Anytime I make my Lasagna (page 163), I make this cashew ricotta to put on each layer of the lasagna, and it comes out amazing every time. I've made this recipe for friends before, and they thought it was actual cow's-milk ricotta! The texture of cashew ricotta is very similar to that of cow's-milk ricotta. The acidity and herbs also add a wonderful balance of flavors to the ricotta.

1 pound raw, unsalted cashews
¼ cup lemon juice
2 garlic cloves, peeled
1 cup unsweetened almond milk
3 tablespoons extra-virgin olive oil
1 tablespoon roughly chopped basil
1 tablespoon roughly chopped Italian parsley
1 tablespoon roughly chopped chives
1½ teaspoons salt
½ teaspoon black pepper

1. Place the cashews in a medium-sized bowl. Pour water into the bowl so the cashews are covered completely. Soak the cashews at least two hours to soften them. After two hours, drain the cashews from the water and transfer them to a food processor.

2. Add all ingredients to the food processor and process until the mixture is completely smooth with no chunks. Transfer the ricotta to an airtight sealed container and refrigerate up to one week.

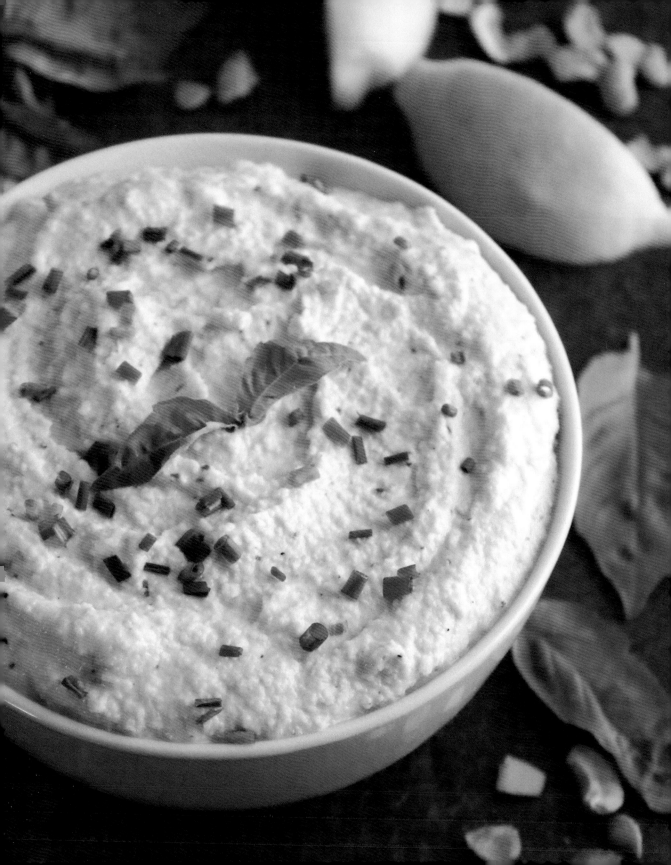

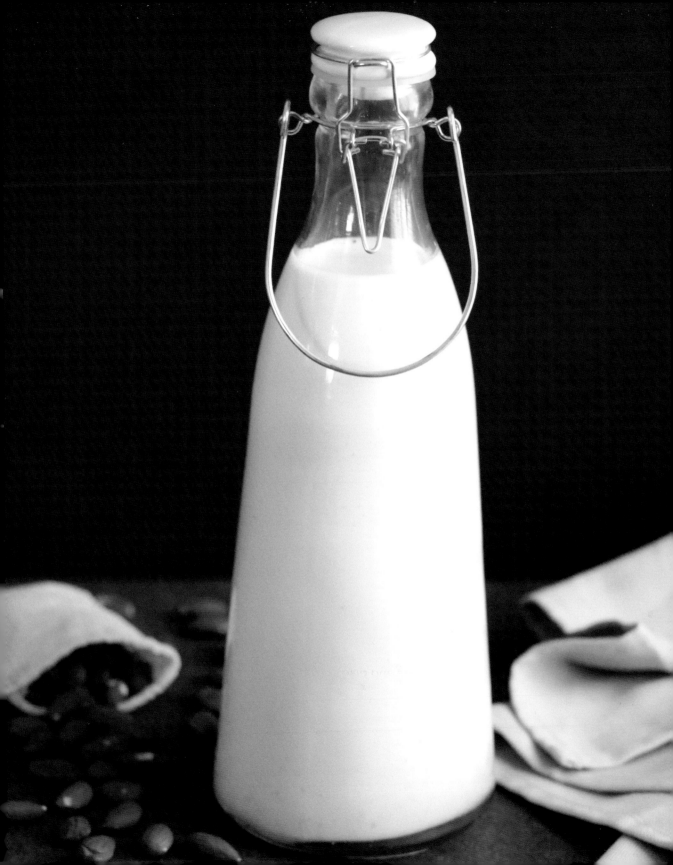

ALMOND MILK

Gluten-Free, Dairy-Free, Grain-Free, Vegan

Yields about 6 Cups

Going dairy-free can be hard at first, but recipes like this almond milk make it so much easier. This almond milk is so creamy and delicious that it's hard to buy store-bought once you've made it yourself. Use this in place of any cow's milk recipe and the results are very similar. My favorite way to use it is poured over granola with fresh bananas and cinnamon.

2 cups raw, unsalted almonds
6 cups filtered water
2 pitted dates
½ teaspoon salt

* You will need a Nut Milk Bag (You can find these at Whole Foods Market or purchase one online)

> **NOTE:** It's normal for homemade almond milk to separate once refrigerated. Just shake it before each use.

1. Soak your almonds in water (just enough water to cover all of the almonds) in a covered container overnight, or at least 12 hours. Drain the almonds from the water and place them in a high-power blender with the 6 cups filtered water. Blend until the mixture is completely smooth.

2. Place a large bowl on a flat surface then pour the almond milk mixture from the blender into the nut milk bag over the bowl. You need to do this in a few batches as you don't want to fill the nut milk bag up too much. Squeeze the milk through the bag into the bowl. Once all liquid is squeezed out of the bag, you can discard the almond meal or save for later use. Repeat these steps until the blender is empty.

3. If the almond milk in the bowl is a bit grainy, you can pour the almond milk through the nut milk bag again into an additional bowl to ensure all the almond meal is removed. Once you've done this, rinse the blender then place the almond milk back in the blender and add in the dates and salt. Blend the almond milk on high speed until the dates are thoroughly combined.

4. Transfer the almond milk to a sealed milk container or mason jars and place in the refrigerator for up to 5 days.

TOMATO SAUCE

Gluten-Free, Dairy-Free, Grain-Free, Vegan

Yields 4–5 Cups

One of my favorite things to make is homemade tomato sauce. I love the fragrance it brings into your kitchen, and it's wonderful to keep in your refrigerator for quick weeknight meals. I've made tomato sauce from fresh tomatoes before, and I've found you can get the same taste results (with much less work) from using canned, crushed tomatoes. This recipe is so fresh, you'll feel as though you should be sitting in a little café in Italy enjoying it with your favorite pasta.

1 cup minced yellow onions
2 tablespoons extra-virgin olive oil
3 (14.5-ounce) cans crushed tomatoes
1 cup canned tomato sauce or tomato puree
5 garlic cloves, minced
⅓ cup roughly chopped fresh basil
⅓ cup roughly chopped Italian parsley
1½ teaspoons salt

1. In a large saucepan or Dutch oven, sauté the onions in olive oil on medium-high heat until translucent. Add in the crushed tomatoes, tomato sauce, garlic, basil, parsley, and salt. Bring the sauce to a boil then reduce the heat to low, cover the pot, and allow the sauce to simmer at least 30 minutes and up to 1 hour.

2. If you prefer your tomato sauce to be more pureed, you can add half the tomato sauce into a food processor once it's done simmering and process it until smooth, then return the sauce back to the pot. I like my tomato sauce slightly chunky so I simply take a potato masher to the sauce to smooth out the bigger chunks of tomato.

3. You can use the tomato sauce right away or let it cool and transfer it to airtight, sealed jars and refrigerate. This sauce tastes even better if you refrigerate it overnight, then use it the next day. The flavors from the sauce soak in and you end up with a richer, heartier tasting tomato sauce.

> **TIP:** When buying crushed tomatoes, it's important to buy high quality tomatoes, preferably from the San Marzano region of Italy. Using quality tomatoes will make the biggest difference in the outcome of your sauce.

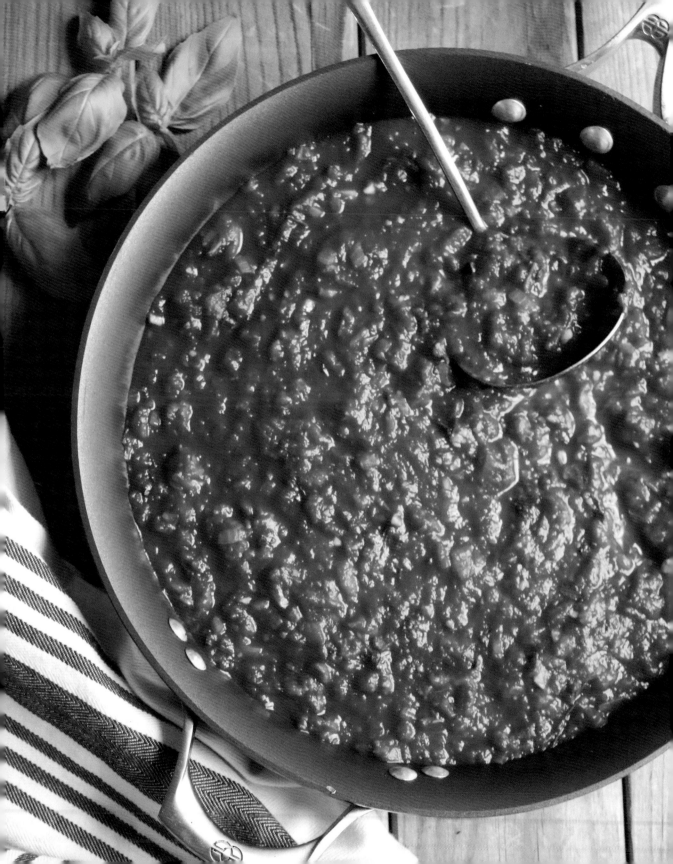

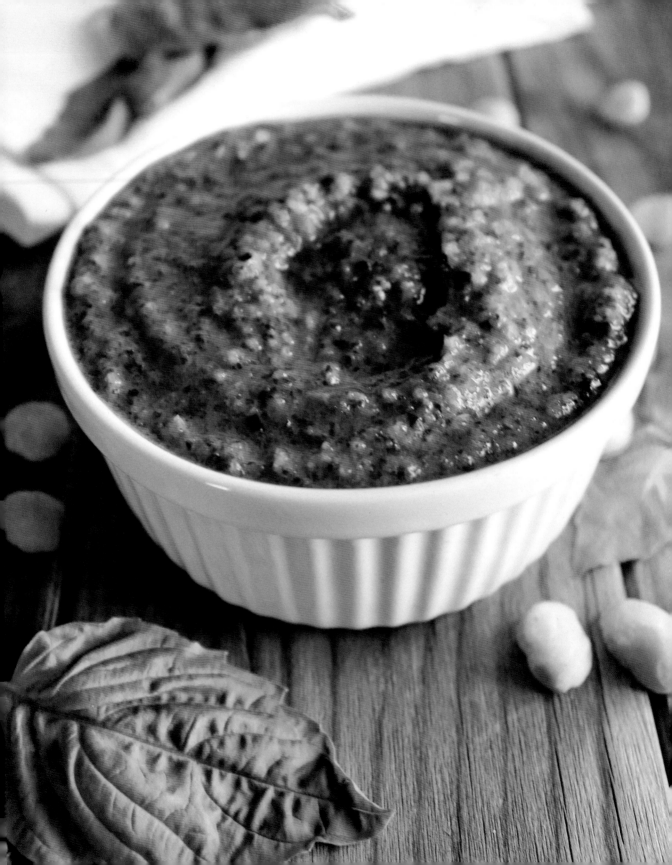

MACADAMIA BASIL PESTO

Gluten-Free, Dairy-Free, Grain-Free, Vegan

Yields about 1 Cup

Pesto is one of those versatile sauces that goes great with just about everything. I love spreading this pesto on top of a white fish and baking it or tossing it over a pasta with chicken. You can even use it as a dip for vegetables! A classic pesto sauce uses pine nuts and Parmesan cheese, but by using macadamia nuts it brings a nutty, buttery, and earthy flavor to the pesto.

1 cup roasted, unsalted whole macadamia nuts
2½ cups packed basil
3 garlic cloves
¾ cup coconut oil
½ teaspoon lemon zest
2 teaspoons lemon juice
½ teaspoon salt
¼ teaspoon black pepper

Place all ingredients in a food processor and process until smooth. Transfer the pesto to a bowl and serve right away or place it in an airtight sealed container and refrigerate up to one week.

ROASTED RED PEPPER HUMMUS

Gluten-Free, Dairy-Free, Vegan

Yields 2½–3 Cups

Hummus is a great healthy snack to have on hand. It's loaded with protein, fiber, and good fat for your heart. I love to make this recipe as an appetizer for friends, served with crisp veggies and rice crackers. Adding the roasted peppers to the hummus is a perfect combination of flavors with the garlic and lemon. You really can eat this stuff by the spoonful!

2 large red bell peppers
½ cup tahini paste
¼ cup lemon juice
¼ cup extra-virgin olive oil
2½ cups cooked or canned garbanzo beans
3 garlic cloves
¼ teaspoon paprika
1 teaspoon salt
¼–½ cup water

1. Line a baking sheet with foil. Place the red peppers on the baking sheet and broil them on high in the middle rack for 15–20 minutes, then flip them over and broil the other side for the same time. The skin will be completely black and charred (don't worry, it peels off). Remove the peppers from the oven and immediately cover them in foil and allow to cool for 15 minutes. Once cooled, slice the tops off and cut the peppers in half, then scoop out the seeds. Peel the charred skin off the peppers. Once all the skin is peeled, dice the peppers and set them aside.

2. In a food processor add the tahini, lemon juice, and olive oil, and process until smooth. Then, add in the garbanzo beans, garlic, paprika, salt, and half the diced red peppers. Begin to process the hummus and from the top opening, add in water until the hummus smoothes out completely.

3. Transfer the hummus to a bowl and top with the remaining half of the roasted peppers and additional paprika. You can serve it immediately or store in the refrigerator up to a week.

> **NOTE:** If you're in a time crunch you can buy store-bought roasted red peppers in a jar instead of roasting them yourself. You will need approximately 2/3 cup of store-bought roasted peppers.

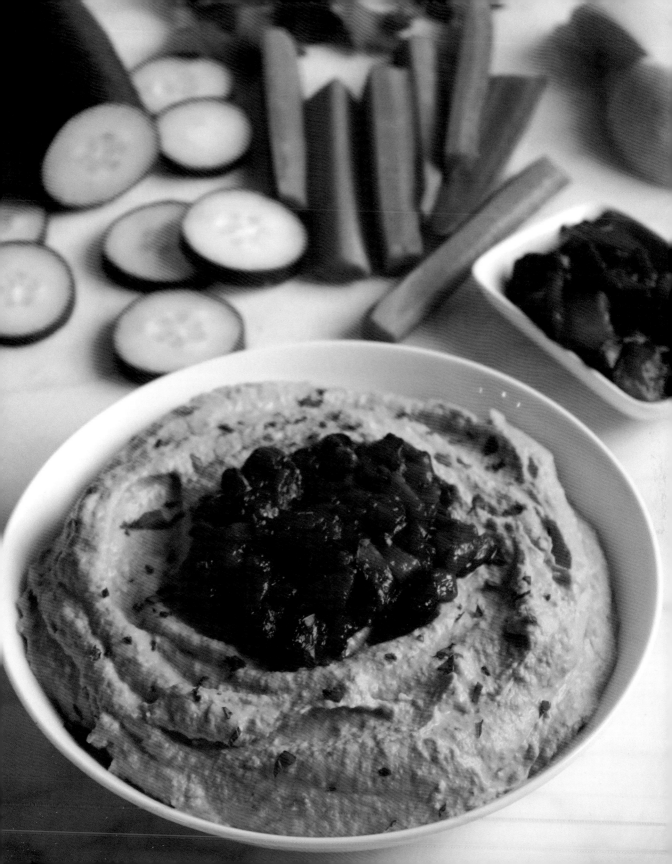

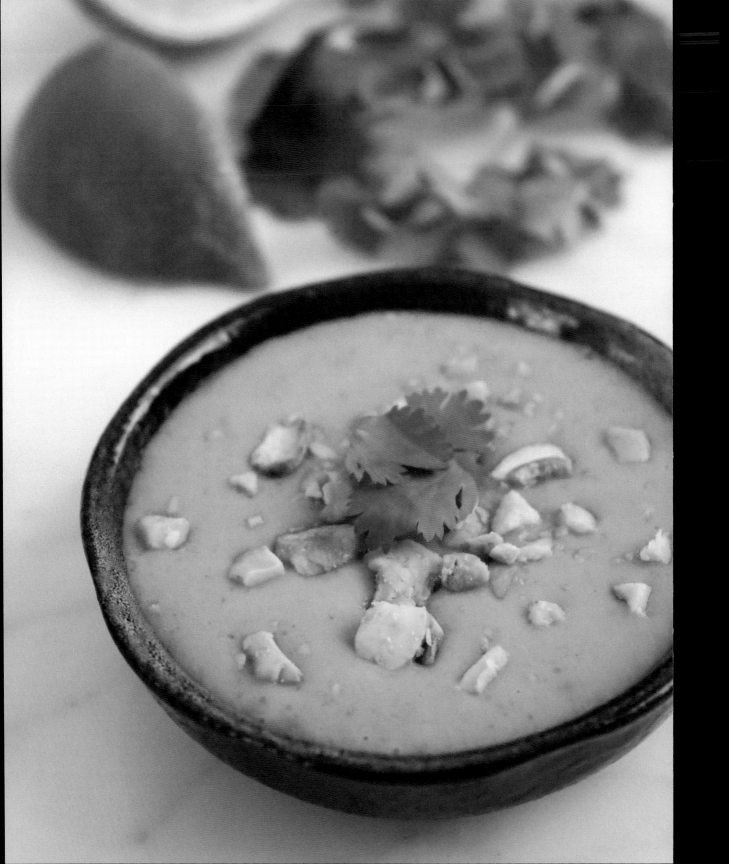

CREAMY PEANUT SAUCE

Gluten-Free, Dairy-Free, Grain-Free, Vegetarian

Yields about ¾ Cup

You'll notice I use this sauce in a lot of my recipes because it's one of those that I make almost every week, and Jason loves this stuff. This sauce goes perfectly with my Rainbow Spring Rolls with Shrimp (page 64), Ground Turkey Asian Lettuce Wraps (page 71), and my Thai Chicken Pizza (page 142). You can even use it as a salad dressing!

3 tablespoons all-natural peanut butter
1 tablespoon lime juice
1–2 tablespoons sriracha (page 128)
1 tablespoon honey
⅓ cup coconut milk
½ teaspoon garlic powder
¼ teaspoon salt
½ teaspoon sesame oil

1. Place all ingredients in a food processor and process until completely smooth. You can store the peanut sauce for up to 2 weeks in the refrigerator.

2. If you refrigerate the sauce it can thicken overnight, so to thin it out, just add a bit more coconut milk or some water.

NOTE: Have you ever tried making homemade peanut butter? It's so stinking easy. Place roasted, unsalted peanuts in a food processor and blend them on high then once the peanut butter gets thick, add in a bit of oil (such as coconut oil) to thin it out and make it smooth. The process only takes a few minutes!

MANGO-MINT SALSA

Gluten-Free, Dairy-Free, Grain-Free, Vegan

Yields 4 Cups

This mango salsa is fantastic over my Blackened Halibut Tacos (see recipe on page 151) or served with corn tortilla chips as a dip. The mango is sweet and you get this lovely acidity from the cherry tomatoes and a fresh bite from the mint.

3 cups diced mango
1 cup diced yellow bell pepper
⅓ cup minced red onion
4 tablespoons minced jalapeños
1 cup cherry tomatoes, sliced in halves
½ cup cilantro
2 tablespoons lime juice
⅓ cup minced mint
½ teaspoon salt
½ teaspoon cumin
½ teaspoon garlic powder

In a medium-sized bowl, mix together all ingredients well. Cover the bowl and place it in the refrigerator for at least an hour before serving. By letting the sauce sit, you really get a more flavorful and better tasting salsa.

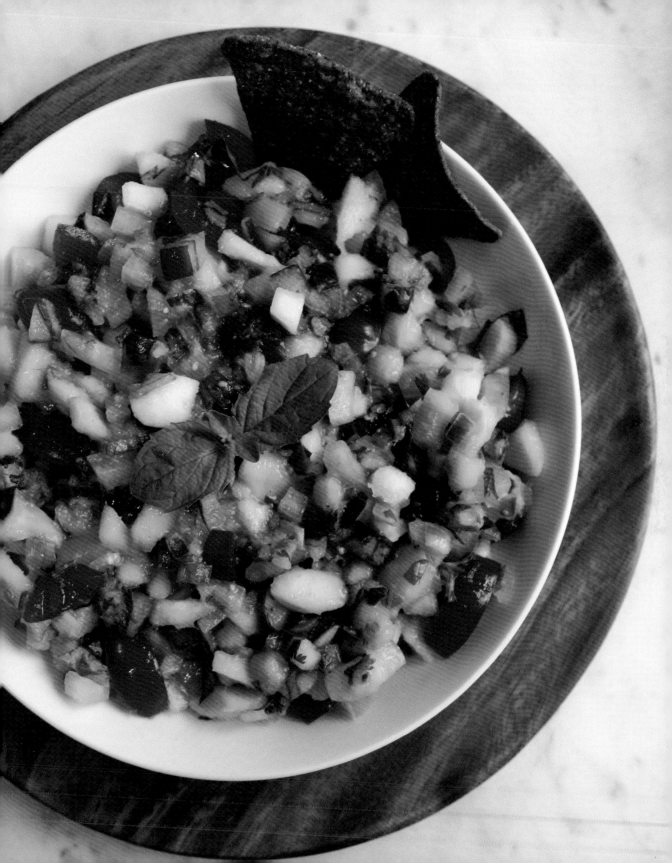

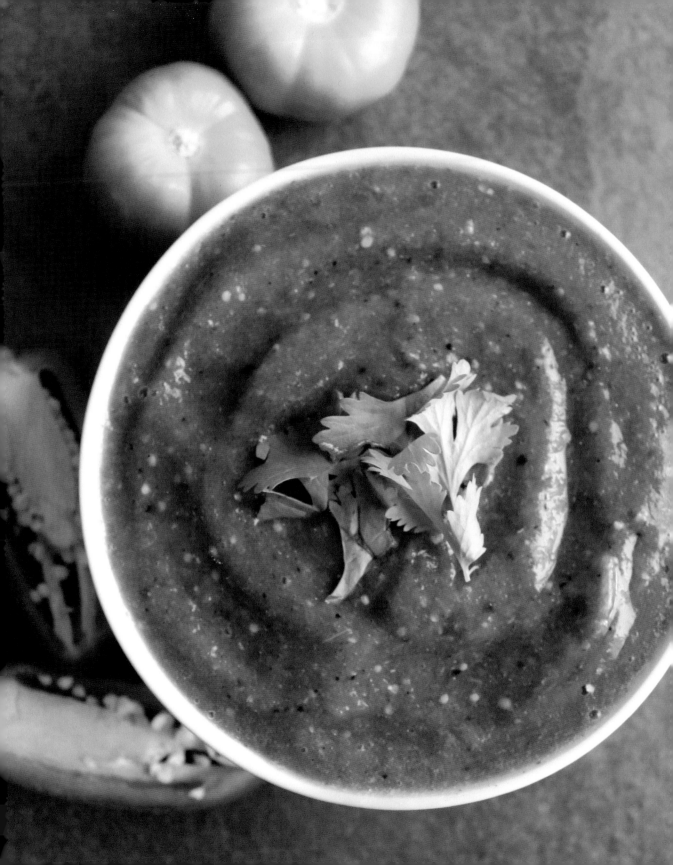

ROASTED TOMATILLO SALSA VERDE

Gluten-Free, Dairy-Free, Grain-Free, Vegan

Yields 2–2½ Cups

This is Jason's favorite salsa I make! He loves it over an omelette for breakfast, tacos for dinner, or to dip veggie sticks in. You get such a deep, intense flavor from roasting the tomatillos first. This salsa can be on the spicier side, so if you don't like the heat, I suggest using only one jalapeño pepper.

12 medium-sized tomatillos, husked
1 yellow onion, skin removed and
  sliced in fourths
1–2 jalapeños, sliced in half
5 garlic cloves, peeled
½ cup minced cilantro
½ teaspoon salt

1. Preheat your oven to 425 degrees.

2. Line a baking sheet with foil then lay down the tomatillos, onions, jalapeños, and garlic cloves. Roast everything for 40 minutes. Remove the baking sheet from the oven and transfer everything into a blender (including the juices from the tomatillos). Blend the salsa on high until completely smooth. Transfer the salsa to a bowl and add in the cilantro and salt. Cover the bowl and allow the salsa to cool for 1 hour in the refrigerator before serving.

> **TIP:** Place the garlic cloves under the onion slices on the baking sheet before roasting. This prevents the garlic from burning and becoming bitter.

SRIRACHA SAUCE

Gluten-Free, Dairy-Free, Grain-Free, Vegan

Yields 1½ Cups

We use sriracha on just about everything! To me, sriracha can take any boring meal to a whole new level. Standard store-bought sriracha sauce is loaded with preservatives and chemicals, so trade in the store-bought version and try making it homemade. You will be pleasantly surprised by how easy it is!

1 pound red jalapeño peppers
½ yellow onion
6 garlic cloves
⅓ cup apple cider vinegar
1 teaspoon grated ginger
1 large pitted date
3 tablespoons coconut aminos
1 teaspoon salt

> **FACT:** The apple cider vinegar acts as a natural preservative, allowing the sriracha sauce to stay fresher longer.

1. Slice the tops off the jalapeños then cut them in half. For a medium-spiced sauce, I scoop half the seeds out of the peppers and leave half in. If you want your sauce super-spicy, you can leave all the seeds in.

2. Place the jalapeños, onions, garlic, apple cider vinegar, ginger, date, coconut aminos, and salt in a high-power blender (not a food processor—it will not puree it enough), and blend on high speed until the sauce is completely smooth.

3. Transfer the sriracha to a saucepan and cook the sauce on medium-high heat for 15–20 minutes. Once the sauce is done, the foam will disappear and the sauce will be a vibrant red color. Transfer the sriracha to an airtight sealed jar and allow it to cool in the refrigerator for one hour before using.

4. The sriracha will stay good in the refrigerator for up to two weeks.

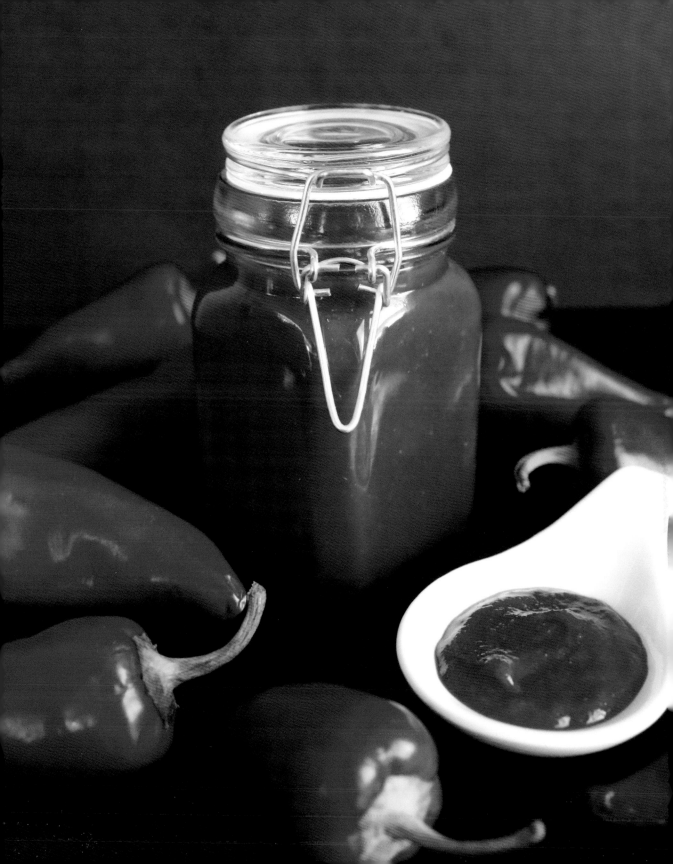

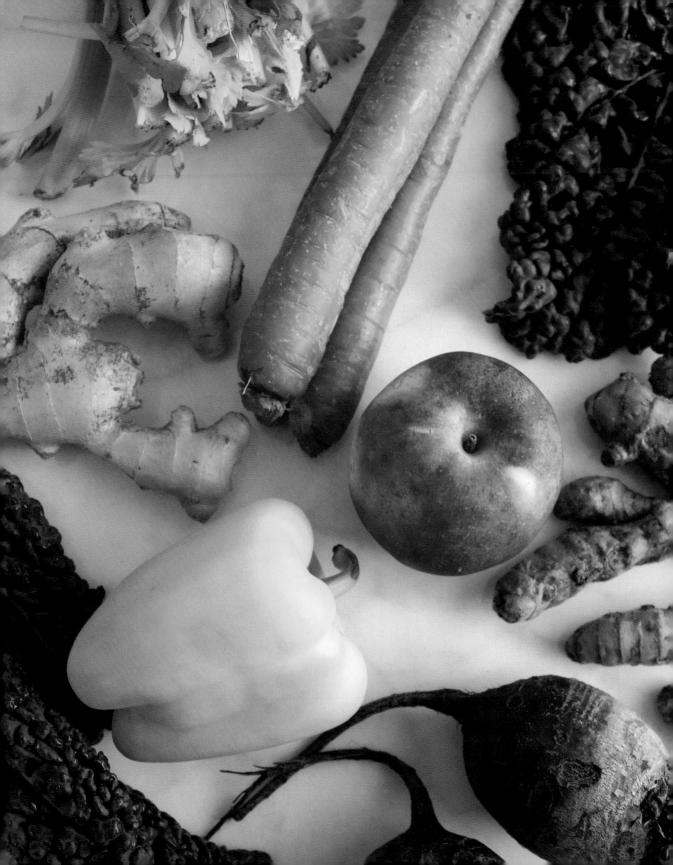

Fresh Juices and Smoothies

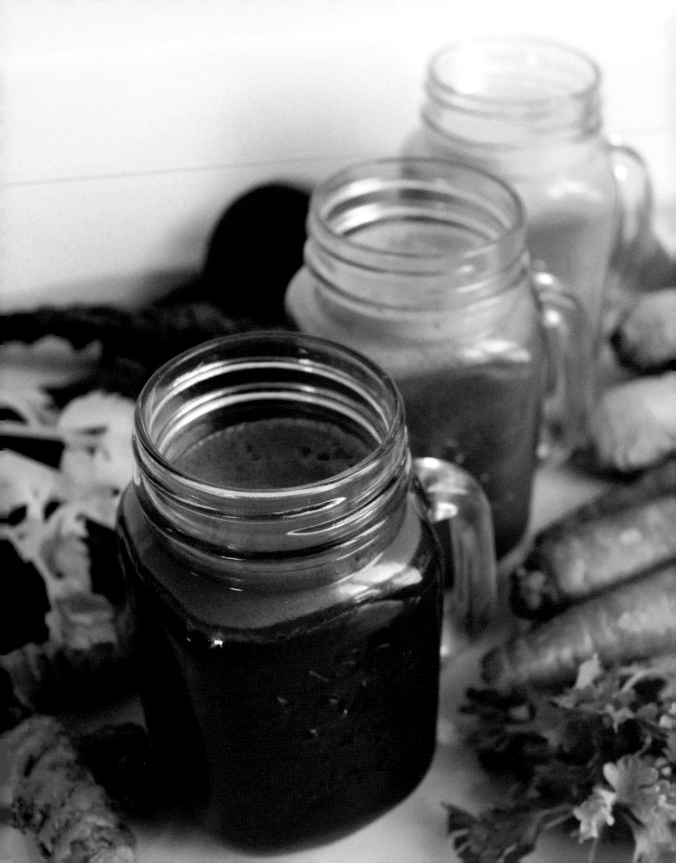

JUICE 3 WAYS

Gluten-Free, Dairy-Free, Grain-Free, Vegan

Yields 16–20 Ounces

Juicing was a huge part of Jason's recovery process. He can be quite selective when it comes to the types of fruits and vegetables he will eat, but if I put them in a juice he will gladly drink it! These are my three favorite juice recipes that are not only so good for detoxing your body and giving it the nutrients it needs, but they actually taste delicious and make you want to drink them.

Pink Juice:
1 large beet
2 celery stalks
2 whole carrots
1 pink lady apple
2–4 inches ginger root (depending on how spicy you prefer it), peeled
½ lemon (juice only)

Green Juice:
2 cucumbers
3 celery stalks
1 green apple
½ lemon (juice only)
1 cup parsley
2–4 inches ginger root, peeled
6 kale leaves

Yellow Juice:
½ medium-large sized pineapple, skin removed
1 yellow bell pepper, stem and seeds removed
1 lemon (juice only)
4 inches turmeric root, peeled

Cut each ingredient so it easily fits through the juicer. Place each ingredient through a juicer, then into a cup or a sealed container. Use only the juice of the lemon, as the peel will make it bitter. It's best to drink the juice immediately, but you can store them in the refrigerator for up to 3 days. It's natural for the juice to separate, so shake each time before use.

> **FACT:** Juicing can boost your immune system with an abundance of vitamins, minerals, and phytonutrients. It also promotes detoxification within your body by ridding it of unwanted toxins, free radicals, and it can help fight against disease.

PITAYA SMOOTHIE BOWL

Gluten-Free, Dairy-Free, Grain-Free, Vegan

Single Serving

Pitaya (a.k.a. dragon fruit) is the fruit of a cactus species. The vibrant pinkish-red color is what you get from the flesh of the fruit, and it's completely natural! One of my favorite breakfasts or lunches to make is this pitaya smoothie bowl. It's incredibly tasty, and leaves you feeling rejuvenated for the entire day.

2 frozen packs unsweetened pitaya puree*
½ frozen banana
⅓ cup frozen mango
½ cup coconut water

Toppings:

Blueberries, raspberries, sliced bananas, mango chunks, and chia seeds, as desired

Place the frozen pitaya packs, banana, mango, and coconut water in a high-power blender and blend until completely smooth and free of chunks. Transfer to a bowl and top with the blueberries, raspberries, banana, mango, and chia seeds.

> **TIP:** You will need a high-power blender for this recipe such as a Vitamix because it has to be able to break through the frozen fruit and puree it. If the blender gets stuck, slap the sides to break the frozen fruit apart.

> ***NOTE:** You can find the frozen packs of unsweetened pitaya in the freezer section with the frozen fruit at most grocery stores.

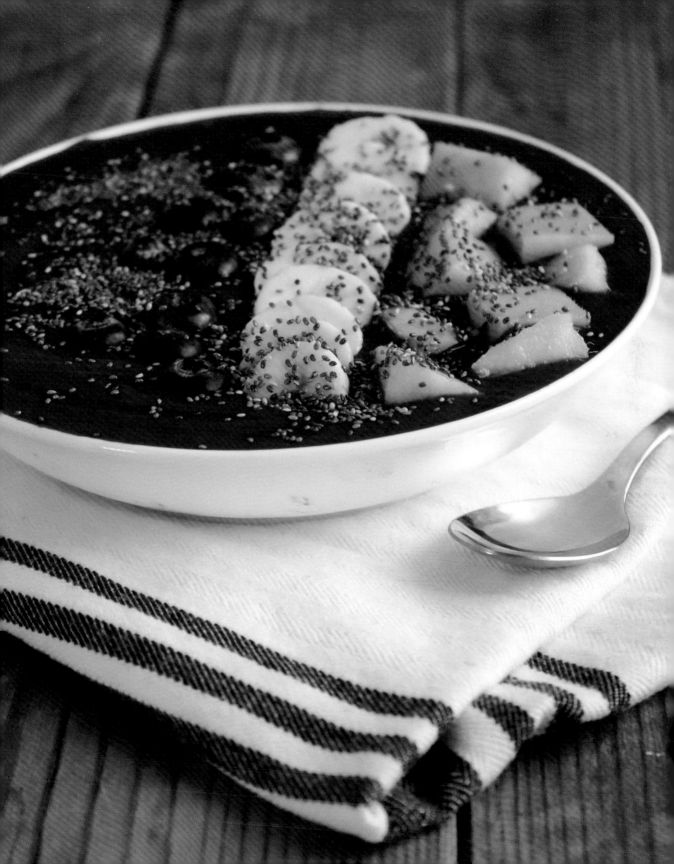

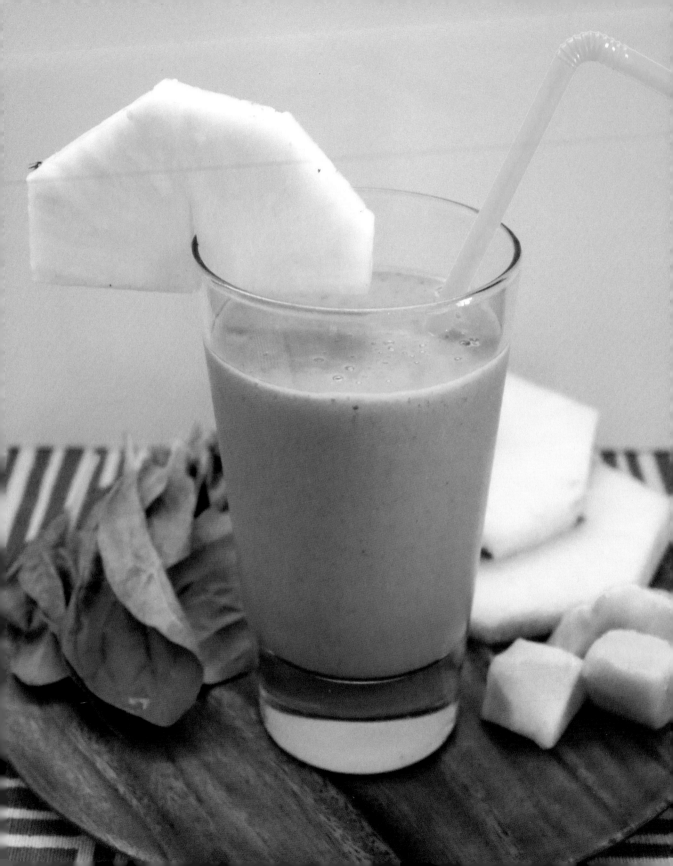

TROPICAL GREEN SMOOTHIE

Gluten-Free, Dairy-Free, Grain-Free, Vegan

Yields about 16 Ounces

This smoothie makes you feel like you're on vacation in the tropics somewhere! It's a great on-the-go smoothie, and not only is it super filling, but it tastes wonderful too.

2 cups packed kale
½ cup packed spinach
1 cup almond milk
1 small banana
¼ cup frozen pineapple chunks
1 teaspoon chia seeds
¼ cup frozen mango chunks
1 inch ginger, peeled and sliced

Place all ingredients in a blender and blend until completely smooth. Transfer the smoothie to a cup and drink it immediately.

TIP: Green smoothies are a perfect way to sneak in kale and spinach for your daily dose of greens! The sweetness from the banana, pineapple, and mango masks the bitterness from the kale and spinach, leaving you with an ultra-delicious, nutrient-packed smoothie!

CHOCOLATE-ALMOND BANANA PROTEIN SMOOTHIE

Gluten-Free, Dairy-Free, Vegan

Yields about 16 Ounces

This smoothie literally tastes like a chocolate-banana milkshake, except it's loaded with protein to help guide you through your day and is packed with nutrients to help your body function at its highest peak. I always make this smoothie for Jason after a workout, or for an easy lunch.

1 scoop chocolate protein powder (see note below)
1 cup almond milk
2 teaspoons almond butter
½ frozen banana
1 teaspoon chia seeds
1 cup ice

Place all ingredients in a blender and blend until completely smooth. Transfer the smoothie to a cup and drink immediately.

> **NOTE:** You have to be careful when buying protein powders and always make sure you check the ingredients label. Most protein powders contain whey, which is a derivative of milk. I always opt for the vegan protein powders to avoid this. The brand I use is Vega and it's gluten-free, dairy-free, with no sugar added, and non-GMO.

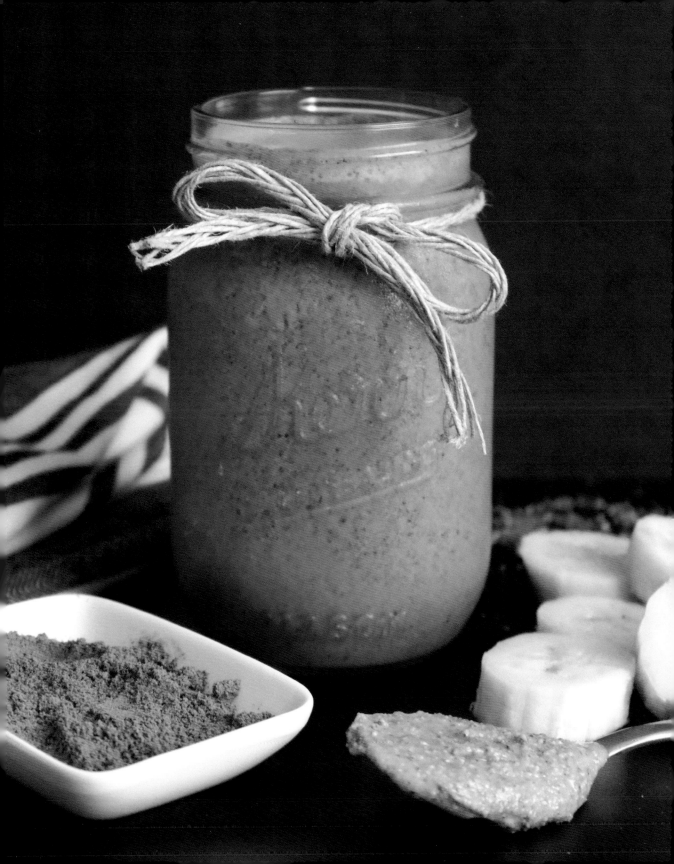

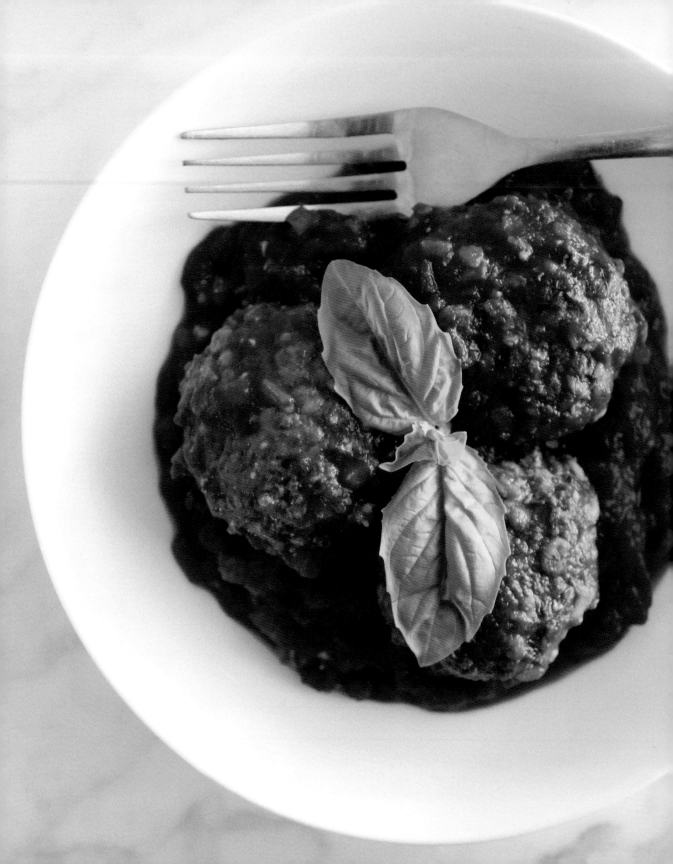

Main Courses

THAI CHICKEN PIZZA

Gluten-Free, Dairy-Free

Serves 2–3

I have an obsession with peanut sauce and this Thai chicken pizza—the perfect combination of sweet and spicy. If you love Thai food and you love pizza, then you are going to love this. There are so many colors, textures, and flavor combinations that make this pizza a must-try recipe.

2 (8–10 inch) gluten-free pizza
   crusts (see note below)
1 diced chicken breast
1 tablespoon extra-virgin olive oil
¼ teaspoon garlic powder
¼ teaspoon black pepper
½ teaspoon salt
4 tablespoons creamy peanut sauce
   (recipe on page 123)

Pizza Toppings:
1 cup shredded purple cabbage
1 whole carrot, shredded
⅓ cup roughly chopped green
   onions
½ cup mung bean sprouts
2 tablespoons minced cilantro
1 tablespoon crushed peanuts
Serve pizzas with lime wedges

1. Preheat your oven to 425 degrees.

2. Cook your pizza crusts according to the package. With most pre-made pizza crusts, you cook the crust a few minutes prior to adding the toppings.

3. In a pan, sauté the chicken in the olive oil, adding in the seasonings. Once the chicken is nearly cooked, turn off the heat and set it aside. The chicken will continue to cook in the oven.

4. To assemble the pizza: Place the pizza crusts on a baking sheet. First, spread half the creamy peanut sauce over each crust. Then top with the chicken, cabbage, carrots, and green onions.

5. Cook the pizzas in the oven about 8–10 minutes, or just until the crust gets crispy.

6. Remove the pizzas from the oven. Now top them with the fresh mung bean sprouts, cilantro, and crushed peanuts. You can also drizzle additional peanut sauce over the pizzas if desired. Slice the pizzas then serve them with lime wedges. These pizzas are also great topped with sriracha.

> **NOTE:** The brand of gluten-free pizza crust I use is Namaste. The pizza comes out perfectly crispy every time.

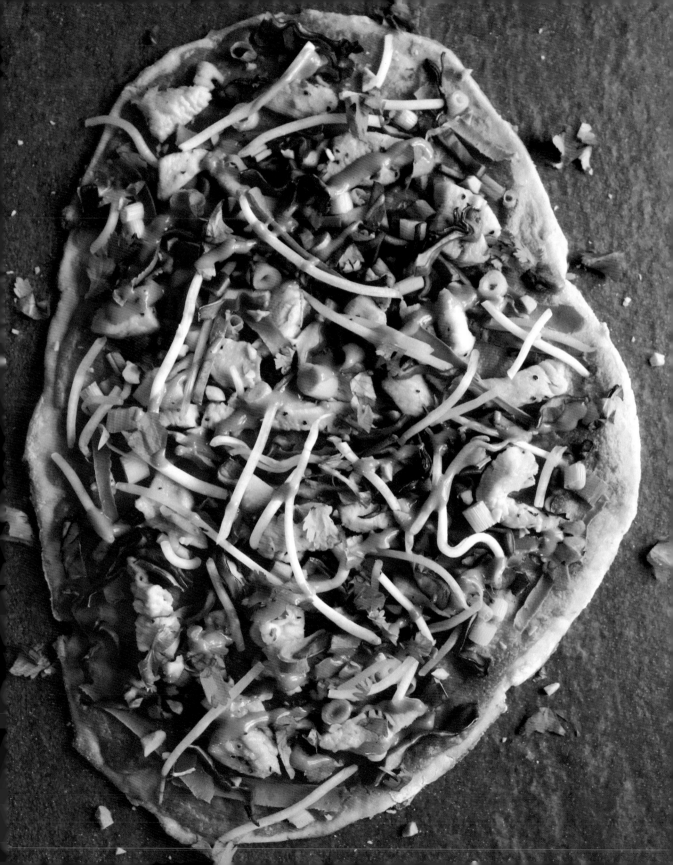

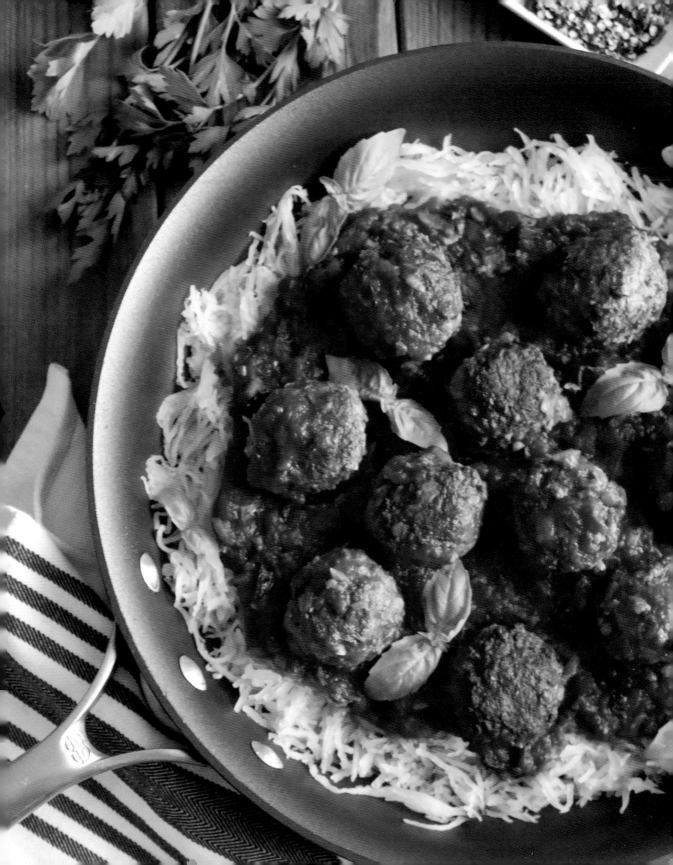

ITALIAN MEATBALLS WITH SPAGHETTI SQUASH

Gluten-Free, Dairy-Free

Serves 4
(Makes 10–12 Meatballs)

Anyone who knows me knows one of my favorite things to make is meatballs, and Jason requests I make this recipe every single week. Traditional Italian meatballs have bread crumbs in them, so in place of bread I use rolled oats, which make the meatballs super tender. These meatballs paired with the spaghetti squash are a home run dinner every time.

For the meatballs:

1 pound ground beef
2 eggs
¾ cup rolled oats
1 tablespoon minced fresh basil
1 tablespoon minced Italian parsley
1 teaspoon garlic powder
½ teaspoon black pepper
1 teaspoon salt
¼ teaspoon crushed red pepper
2 tablespoons extra-virgin olive oil

3–4 pound spaghetti squash
4 cups tomato sauce*,**
Fresh minced basil, to top

1. Preheat oven to 400 degrees. Slice spaghetti squash in half and scoop out the seeds. Brush the tops of the squash in olive oil then lay them face down on a baking sheet. Bake for 45–60 minutes.

2. Prepare the meatballs. In a bowl, combine all meatball ingredients together with your hands. Form the mixture into 10–12 equally sized meatballs. In a large saucepan or Dutch oven, heat the olive oil. Add meatballs to the pan, frying them for 1–2 minutes on each side or until golden brown.

* If you are going to make my tomato sauce recipe (page 116), remove meatballs from the Dutch oven and use the oil/drippings from the meatballs (this adds so much flavor) to saute the onions. Once the sauce is made, add the meatballs back into the Dutch oven with the tomato sauce.

** If you are not making the tomato sauce, you can use a good quality store-bought tomato sauce. After you fry the meatballs on each side, simply pour 4 cups of tomato sauce into the Dutch oven.

Simmer the sauce, covered on low for 30 minutes or until cooked through.

3. Once the squash is done cooking, remove from the oven and allow it to cool for a few minutes. Using a fork, gently scrape the spaghetti squash out of the skin. Serve topped with the tomato sauce, meatballs, and fresh basil.

CHILI-RUBBED RIB EYE STEAK WITH CHIMICHURRI AND ROASTED POTATO WEDGES

Gluten-Free, Dairy-Free, Grain-Free

2–3 Servings

Chimichurri is garlicky sauce from Argentina and is typically served with grilled meats. I love making this recipe for date night in! The chili-rubbed rib eye is so flavorful and juicy and is perfectly complemented by the tangy chimichurri sauce.

1 teaspoon chili powder
½ teaspoon cumin
¼ teaspoon garlic powder
¼ teaspoon salt
¼ teaspoon black pepper
1 pound rib eye steak

Roasted Potato Wedges:

1 large russet potato, sliced
    lengthwise into wedges
2 tablespoons extra-virgin olive oil
1 teaspoon minced fresh thyme
½ teaspoon salt

Chimichurri Sauce:

1 cup roughly chopped cilantro
1 cup roughly chopped Italian parsley
½ cup roughly chopped basil
½ cup extra-virgin olive oil
2 tablespoons apple cider vinegar
1 teaspoon honey
½ lime, juiced
3 garlic cloves
½ teaspoon crushed red pepper
½ teaspoon black pepper
½ teaspoon salt

1. Preheat your oven to 425 degrees.

2. In a small bowl, mix together the chili powder, cumin, garlic powder, salt, and pepper. Generously season each side of the steak, patting the seasoning on and making sure it sticks. We prefer to barbeque the steak on the grill, but you could also use a skillet and it will come out just as well. Grill the steaks at 450 degrees for 6–7 minutes on each side. The cooking time will vary depending on the thickness in the cut of the rib eye.

3. Toss the potato wedges in the olive oil, thyme, and salt. On a greased baking sheet, lay each potato wedge down, being careful not to overcrowd or let them touch. Bake the potatoes for 15 minutes, then flip them over and bake the other side for 10–15 more minutes or until the potatoes are cooked through and crispy.

4. For the chimichurri sauce, place all ingredients in a food processor and process until smooth. Transfer to a bowl.

5. After the steak is done grilling, allow it to rest at least 5–10 minutes. Once it's rested, slice the rib eye into pieces. Serve the steak topped with the chimichurri sauce and a side of the roasted potato wedges.

> **NOTE:** This chimichurri sauce recipe makes a large portion so save it for meals throughout the week. It's great over some grilled chicken or fish!

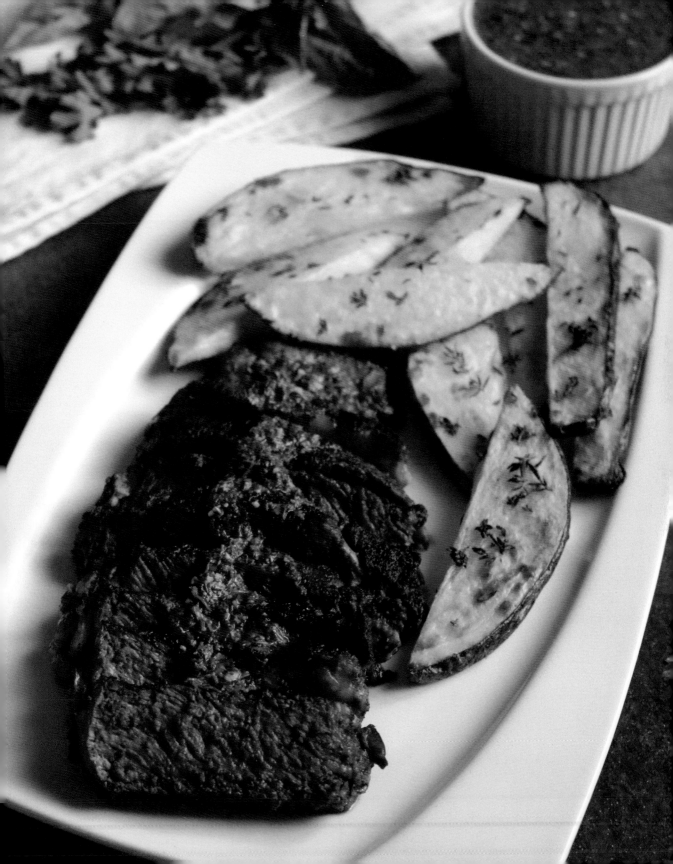

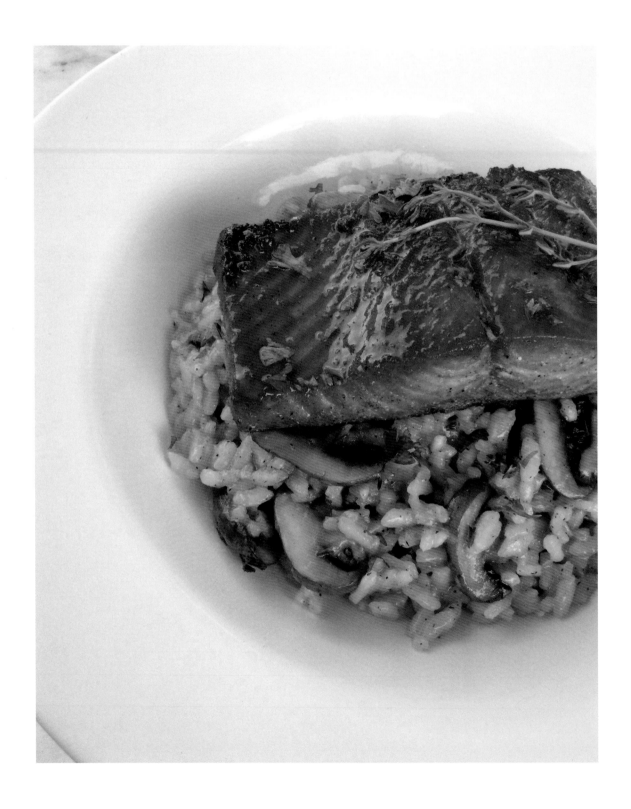

SWEET AND SPICY SALMON WITH MUSHROOM RISOTTO

Gluten-Free, Dairy-Free

2 Servings

This is my go-to foolproof salmon recipe, and there is nothing more comforting than a good risotto. Risotto is a labor of love, but the outcome is always spectacular. It's an Italian dish made from Arborio rice that is cooked slowly in broth to give it that creamy consistency. This mushroom risotto in combination with the sweet and spicy glazed salmon is sure to be your new favorite weeknight recipe.

½ lemon, juiced
1 tablespoon extra-virgin olive oil
1 tablespoon + 1 teaspoon honey
1 teaspoon minced Italian parsley
½ teaspoon garlic powder
½ teaspoon onion powder
¼ teaspoon paprika
½ teaspoon salt
¼ teaspoon black pepper
¼ teaspoon cayenne pepper
1 pound wild-caught salmon filets

Mushroom Risotto:

2 shallots, minced
4 large garlic cloves, minced
2 tablespoons extra-virgin olive oil
2 cups thinly sliced mushrooms
1 teaspoon minced thyme
1 cup Arborio rice
3½ cups low-sodium chicken broth
    (at room temperature or warmed)
3 tablespoons full-fat coconut milk
½ teaspoon salt
½ teaspoon black pepper

1. For the salmon, combine the lemon juice, olive oil, honey, parsley, and seasonings in a bowl. Place the salmon filets in a large plastic bag and pour the marinade in the bag over the salmon. Let the salmon marinate for 30–60 minutes.

2. Preheat your oven to 425 degrees. Line a baking sheet with foil then lay your salmon on top and pour whatever marinade is left in the bag over the top of the salmon. Bake for 10–12 minutes.*

3. For the mushroom risotto, sauté the shallots and garlic in olive oil in a skillet until the shallots are translucent. Add in the mushrooms and thyme and continue to sauté until the mushrooms have softened. Add in the rice and stir quickly until the rice is well-coated.

4. Reduce the heat to medium-low and add in ½ cup of chicken broth. Once the liquid absorbs into the rice, continue to add in the broth ½ cup at a time. The risotto should be slightly firm, yet creamy but not mushy, and that's when it is ready. This process should take about 15–20 minutes.

5. Lastly, add in the coconut milk, salt, and pepper and stir until everything is well combined. Adding the coconut milk at the end adds an extra creaminess without making the risotto too mushy. Serve the salmon on top of the mushroom risotto.

TIP: For perfectly baked salmon, bake the salmon for 4–6 minutes for every ½ inch of thickness in salmon.

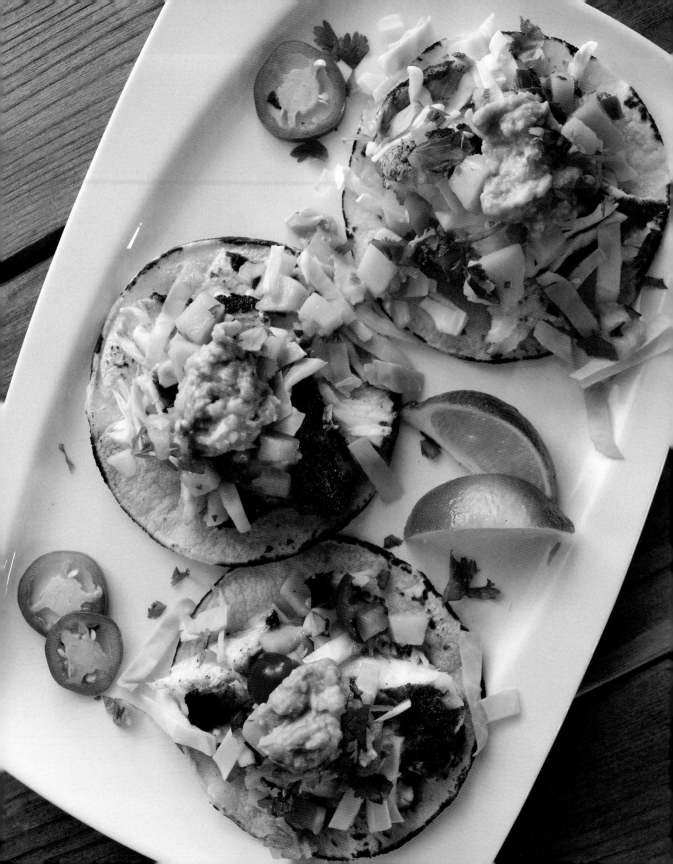

BLACKENED HALIBUT TACOS

Gluten-Free, Dairy-Free

Makes about 8–10 Tacos

One of my favorite ways to use halibut is making tacos. I always make these tacos when I don't feel like cooking a fancy dinner, and they are so delicious during warm summer nights topped with mango-mint salsa (page 124).

Blackened Halibut:

½ teaspoon paprika
½ teaspoon chili powder
½ teaspoon salt
¼ teaspoon black pepper
½ teaspoon garlic powder
¾ pound wild-caught halibut
1½ tablespoons extra-virgin
   olive oil

1 large avocado, smashed
¼ teaspoon salt
½ lime, juiced
8–10 mini corn tortillas
2 cups shredded green cabbage
Lime wedges

*Serve topped with mango-mint
   salsa (page 124)*

1. For the fish, in a small bowl combine the paprika, chili powder, salt, black pepper, and garlic powder. Generously season each side of the halibut with the seasoning.

2. Mix together the avocado, salt, and lime, and set aside.

3. Heat a skillet on medium-high and add in the olive oil. Sear each side of the fish for 4–5 minutes, depending on the thickness of the filet. As the fish is cooking, warm each corn tortilla on a stove-top burner 10–15 seconds on each side.

4. Once the halibut is cooked through, gently break it apart with a fork into pieces. To assemble the tacos, lay a corn tortilla down then top with the blackened halibut, shredded cabbage, guacamole, and mango-mint salsa, and squeeze lime juice over each taco.

COCONUT CHICKEN CURRY

Gluten-Free, Dairy-Free, Grain-Free

Serves 3–4

Jason craves chicken curry, and I make this recipe all the time. There is something so warm and soothing about curry. You can find curry powder at any grocery store, and it's a seasoning made up with fragrant ingredients like turmeric, coriander, and ginger. What I love about curry is that it's not only made up of so many healing ingredients, but it's a one-pot dish and requires no skill level whatsoever.

2 chicken breasts, cubed
2 tablespoons extra-virgin olive oil
2 (15-ounce) cans coconut milk
2 cups thinly sliced mushrooms
4 garlic cloves, minced
½ tablespoon grated ginger
1 red jalapeño, sliced thin
⅓ cup roughly chopped basil
⅓ cup roughly chopped cilantro
½ cup green onions
4–5 tablespoons yellow curry powder
1 tablespoon honey
½ teaspoon salt
1 large russet potato, cubed
½–1 cup low-sodium chicken broth (optional)

Serve with a side of brown rice or cauliflower rice

1. In a Dutch oven or large saucepan, sauté the chicken in the olive oil until cooked. Remove the chicken from the pot and set it aside. Add in the coconut milk, mushrooms, garlic, ginger, jalapeños, basil, cilantro, green onions, curry powder, honey, and salt. Bring the curry to a boil, then reduce the heat to low and let it simmer for at least 30 minutes and up to 1 hour.

2. Turn the heat to medium-high and add in the potatoes. Cover the pot and cook the potatoes 15–20 minutes in the curry sauce, or until they are fork tender. Add the cooked chicken back into the curry. If you want to thin the curry sauce out, you can add in the chicken broth.

3. Serve the curry topped with additional fresh cilantro, basil, and with a side of rice.

> **FACT:** Turmeric (which is one of the main ingredients in curry powder) is one of the most healing foods on the planet. Turmeric is a proven and powerful anti-inflammatory and helps to fight inflammation in our system, where disease breeds.

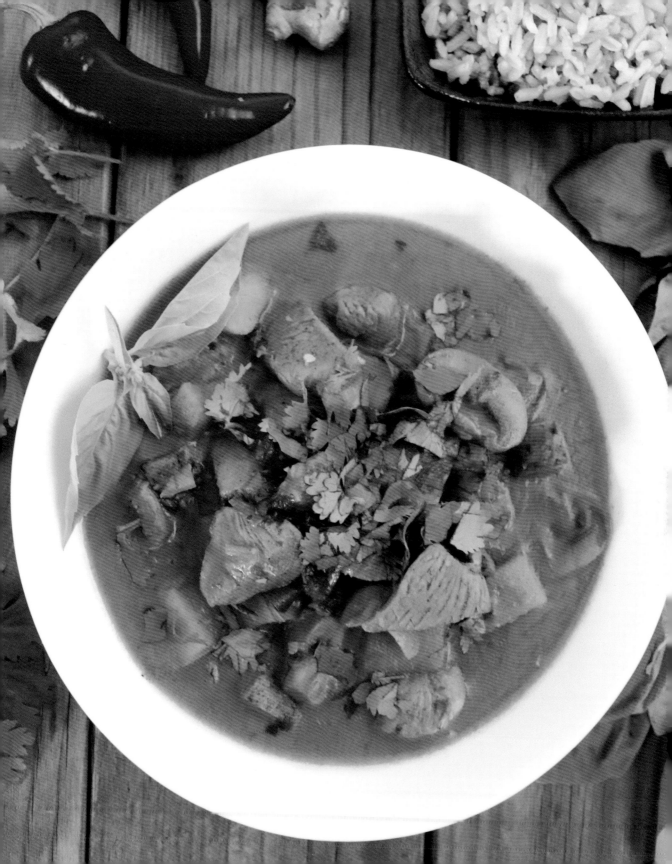

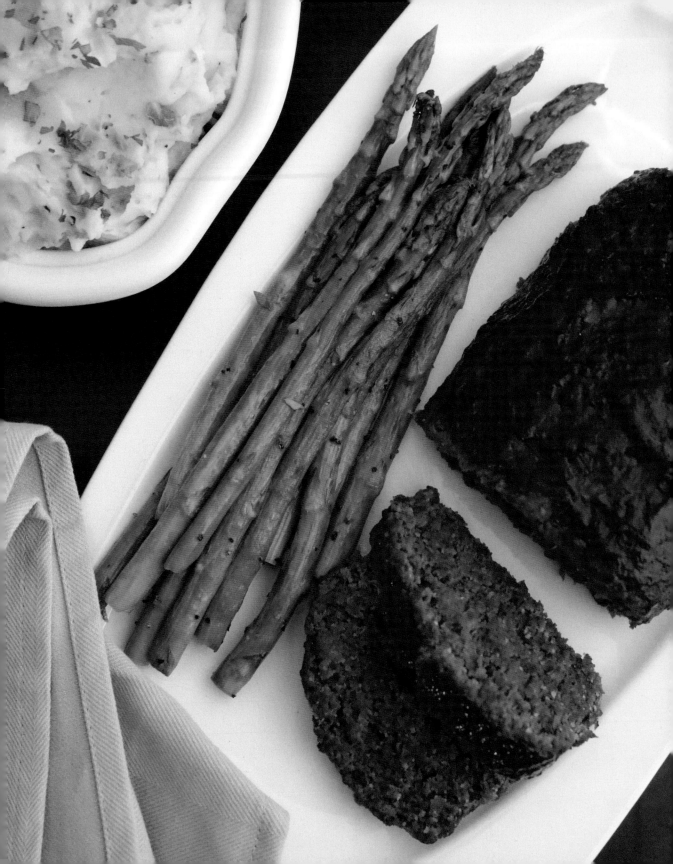

MEATLOAF WITH MASHED POTATOES

Gluten-Free, Dairy-Free

2–3 Servings

You'll never need another meatloaf recipe after making this one. This meatloaf is made gluten-free by using rolled oats in place of traditional bread crumbs. Jason used to hate meatloaf growing up, but I won him over once he tried my version. I use this mashed potatoes recipe all the time—you would never know they are dairy-free and secretly healthy!

Meatloaf:

1 pound ground beef
¾ cup rolled oats
2 eggs
⅓ cup ketchup
1 tablespoon Worcestershire sauce
2 tablespoons minced Italian parsley
5 large basil leaves, minced
1 teaspoon garlic powder
1 teaspoon onion powder
½ teaspoon salt
½ teaspoon black pepper

Topping:

3 tablespoons ketchup

Mashed Potatoes:

4 russet potatoes, cut in half
1¼ cup full-fat coconut milk
1 teaspoon minced thyme
1 teaspoon garlic powder
1 teaspoon salt
¼ teaspoon black pepper
Minced Italian parsley, to top

1. Preheat your oven to 375 degrees.

2. In a large bowl, mix together all meatloaf ingredients well. Spray a baking sheet with a non-stick cooking spray and transfer meatloaf mixture onto the baking sheet. Form the mixture into a meatloaf shape with your hands (you can also use a loaf pan, but I prefer to mold it myself). Bake the meatloaf uncovered for 30 minutes. Remove the meatloaf from the oven and evenly spread the ketchup on top. Return to the oven and bake an additional 15 minutes. Let the meatloaf stand for 10 minutes before slicing and serving.

3. For the mashed potatoes, bring a pot of water to a boil then add in the potatoes. Boil for 15–20 minutes or until the potatoes are cooked through and fork tender. Drain the boiled potatoes from the water and transfer them to a bowl. Gently smash the potatoes down, then using an electric hand mixer, add in the coconut milk ¼ cup at a time until the potatoes are smooth and creamy with no chunks. Lastly, add in the seasonings to the mashed potatoes. Top with fresh, minced parsley. Serve the meatloaf sliced with a side of mashed potatoes.

GRILLED HAWAIIAN PORTOBELLO MUSHROOM BURGERS WITH TERIYAKI SAUCE

Gluten-Free, Dairy-Free, Grain-Free

2 Servings

Yes, you can use Portobello mushroom caps in place of bread for burgers! Not only are Portobello mushrooms the perfect size for burgers, but they add tons of flavor and texture. This burger is a sweet and savory dream with the grilled pineapple, onions, and homemade (clean) teriyaki sauce.

4 large Portobello mushroom caps
2 tablespoons extra-virgin olive oil
½ sweet onion, sliced in medium-
    thick rings
2 pineapple slices, cored
2 ground beef burger patties,
    seasoned with salt and pepper
Iceberg lettuce, as desired

Teriyaki Sauce:

3 tablespoons coconut aminos
1 tablespoon honey
1 tablespoon apple cider vinegar
1 garlic clove, minced
¼ teaspoon crushed red pepper

> **TIP:** If you like extra sauce on your burgers, I recommended doubling the recipe for the teriyaki sauce. It's finger-licking good.

1. Heat your grill to 400 degrees.

2. For the teriyaki sauce, place all ingredients in a small saucepan. Bring the sauce to a rapid boil, whisking it constantly until the sauce begins to thicken. Reduce the heat to low and let the sauce simmer while you start on the grill.

3. For the Portobello mushrooms, first remove the stem, then remove the black gills. To remove the gills, start from the center of the mushroom and scoop them out with a spoon. These mushrooms can be fragile and can break, so scoop gently. Brush the tops and bottoms of the mushrooms with olive oil. With the top facing down, grill the mushrooms for 5–6 minutes directly on the grill. If excess moisture comes out of the mushroom caps, just soak it up with a paper towel.

4. Lightly grease the grill grates. Grill the onions and pineapples on each side for 3–4 minutes or until blackened grill marks appear. Grill your burger patties for 8–10 minutes, depending on your preferred temperature.

5. To assemble the burgers, start with a mushroom cap then layer it with the beef patty, teriyaki sauce, onions, pineapple, lettuce, and top it all with another mushroom cap.

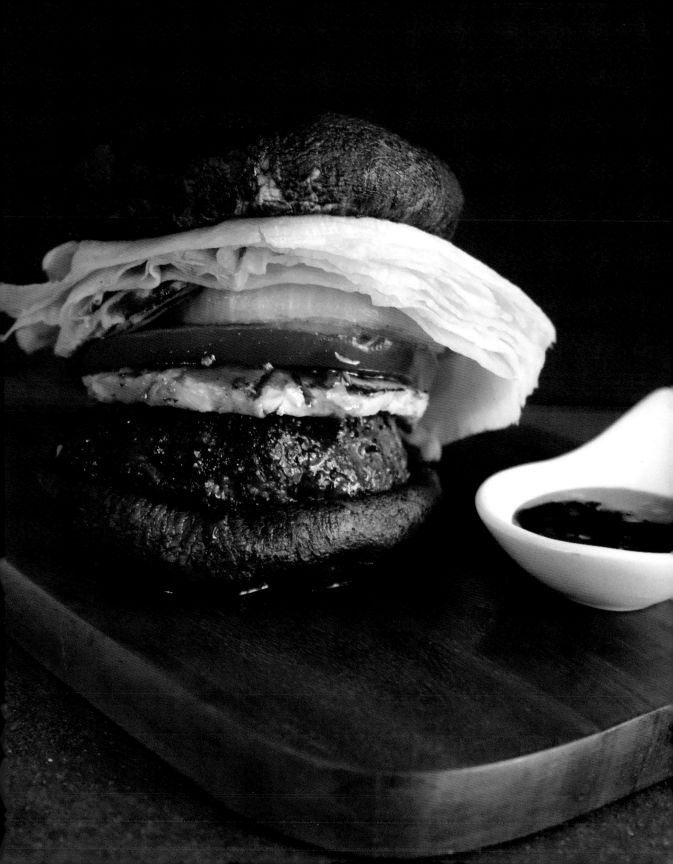

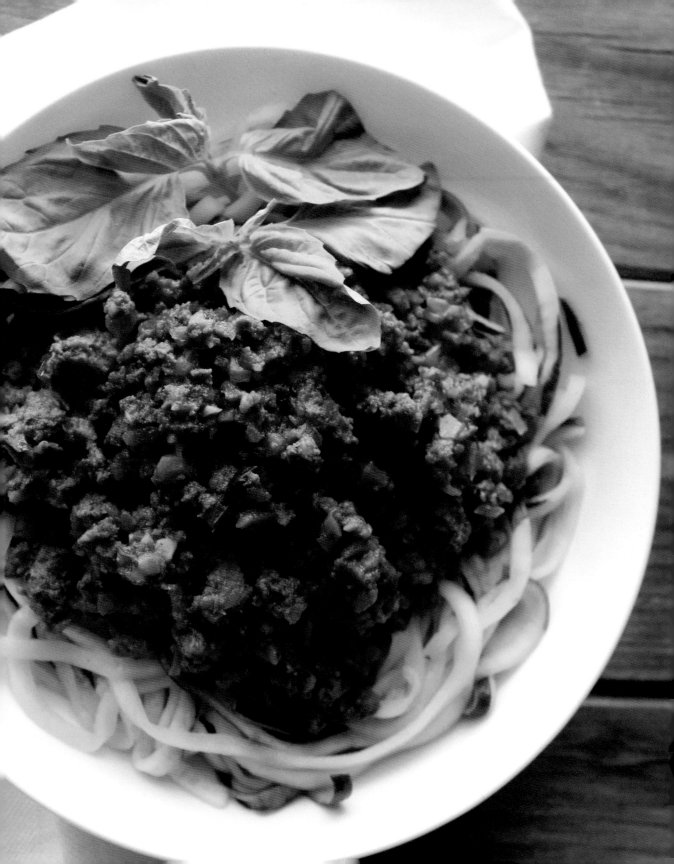

BOLOGNESE WITH ZUCCHINI NOODLES

Gluten-Free, Dairy-Free, Grain-Free

4 Servings

This simple Bolognese sauce is an Italian classic. The key to a good Bolognese is allowing the sauce to simmer slowly on low heat to make the beef tender, and to allow all the flavors from the vegetables and herbs come out. This meaty Bolognese recipe is lightened up with zucchini noodles for a very satisfying and easy weeknight dinner.

Bolognese:

3 tablespoons extra-virgin olive oil
½ yellow onion, minced
2 whole carrots, finely chopped
2 celery stalks, finely chopped
¾ cup dry white wine (optional)
½ cup low-sodium chicken broth
3 garlic cloves, minced
1 pound ground beef
½ pound spicy Italian chicken
    sausage
3 tablespoons tomato paste
6 large basil leaves, roughly
    chopped
1 tablespoon minced Italian parsley
1 teaspoon black pepper
1½ teaspoons salt
½ cup unsweetened almond milk

Zucchini Noodles:

6 medium-large zucchinis,
    spiralized
1 tablespoon extra-virgin olive oil
Fresh minced basil, to top
Crushed red pepper, to top

1. In a Dutch oven or a large saucepan, add in 2 tablespoons of olive oil, the onions, carrots, and celery. Sauté the mirepoix a few minutes until the onions are translucent. Add in the white wine, chicken broth, and garlic, and simmer on medium heat until the liquid reduces by half.

2. In a skillet, add in 1 tablespoon of olive oil along with the ground beef and chicken sausage. Break apart the meats with a spatula and sauté until the meat is fully cooked and browned. Add the meat into the Dutch oven.

3. Then, add in the tomato paste, basil, parsley, black pepper, salt, and ¼ cup of the almond milk, mixing everything together well. Cover the pot and let the Bolognese simmer on low heat for at least 30 minutes and up to 2 hours, stirring it every so often. For a creamier Bolognese sauce, add in the remaining almond milk.

4. For the zucchini noodles, sauté them in a skillet with 1 table-spoon of olive oil on medium-high heat. The zucchini noodles will cook fast, in about 2–4 minutes, so be careful not to over-cook them. If excess water comes out of the zucchini noodles, you can strain them before serving.

5. Serve the zucchini noodles topped with the Bolognese, fresh basil, and crushed red pepper for added spice.

BUFFALO CHICKEN AND QUINOA STUFFED PEPPERS

1-Free, Dairy-Free

2 Servings

I've always loved stuffed peppers so I decided to put a twist on the traditional stuffed pepper recipe by adding in buffalo chicken and quinoa. Quinoa is one of the most protein-rich foods we can eat, and is loaded with fiber. This dish is so colorful and absolutely scrumptious.

4 large multi-colored bell peppers
3 tablespoons coconut oil
1 cup yellow onions, minced
4 garlic cloves, minced
2 cups shredded cooked chicken
1½ cups white quinoa, cooked
⅓ cup buffalo sauce
Dash of black pepper
1 large avocado, diced
1 tablespoon minced cilantro

Serve with additional buffalo sauce, to top

1. Preheat your oven to 425 degrees.

2. Cut the tops off the bell peppers, scoop out the seeds, then brush the peppers in 2 tablespoons of coconut oil. Place the bell peppers (cut side up) in a small casserole dish. Fill the bottom of the casserole dish ¼ of the way with water, cover the dish in foil, and bake the peppers for 20 minutes. Remove the peppers from the oven and use a paper towel to soak up the liquid that forms inside of each pepper.

3. In a skillet, sauté the onions and garlic in 1 tablespoon of coconut oil until the onions are translucent. Transfer to a large bowl. In the bowl, add in the cooked chicken, quinoa, buffalo sauce, and black pepper. Stuff each pepper equally with the filling, cover the dish with foil, and bake an additional 20–25 minutes. Remove the peppers from the oven and top them with diced avocado and cilantro, and drizzle more buffalo sauce over the tops.

> *TIP:* I use the Frank's RedHot brand for the buffalo sauce—it's all-natural and absolutely delicious.

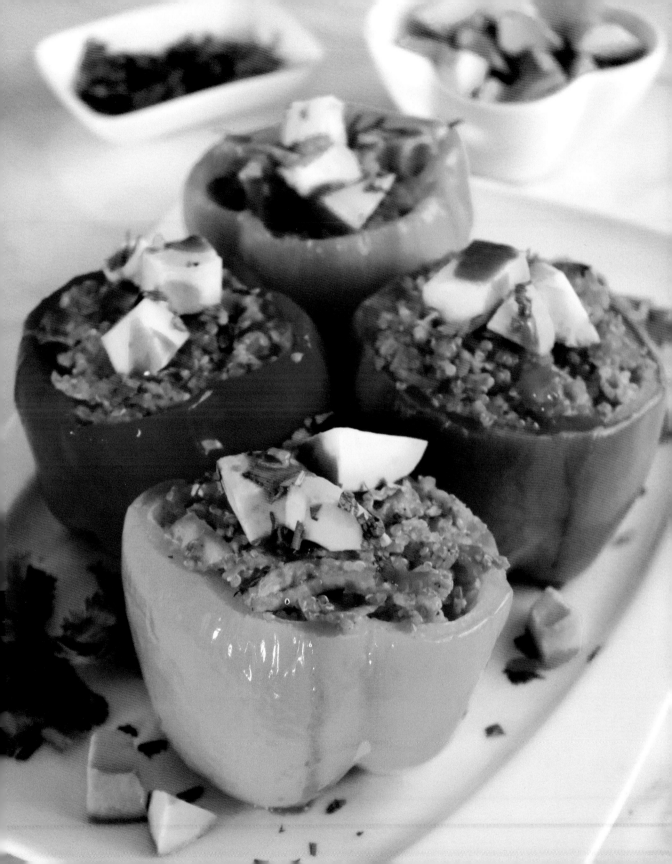

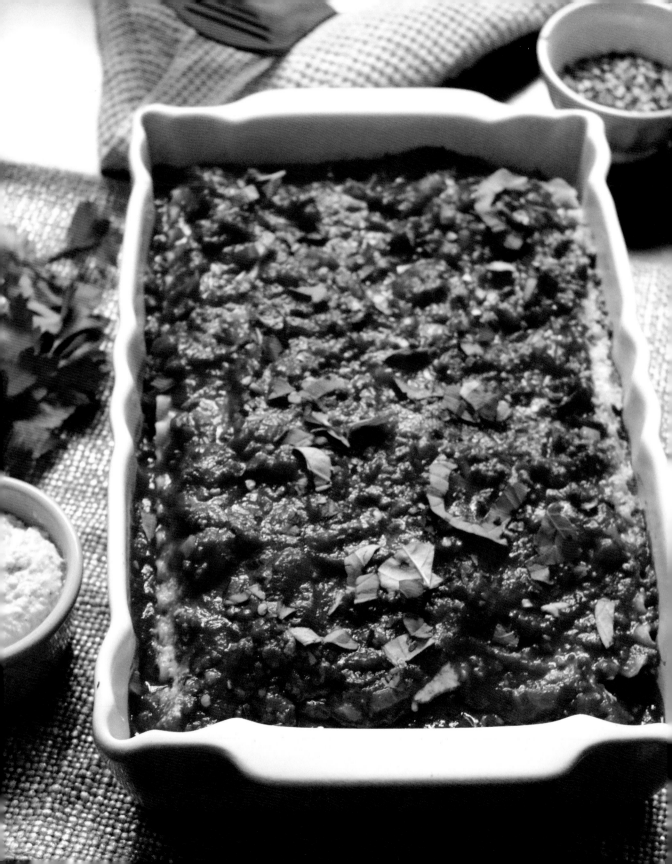

LASAGNA

Gluten-Free, Dairy-Free

4–6 Servings

Jason has always loved lasagna ever since he was little. So once he went gluten- and dairy-free, lasagna seemed like it would forever be on the no-no list. I decided to come up with a way to make him a healthy lasagna that he could actually eat and not get sick from—mission accomplished! This lasagna is so comforting, luscious, and has become a family favorite.

Meat Sauce:

1 cup minced yellow onions
2 tablespoons extra-virgin olive oil
1 pound ground beef
5 garlic cloves, minced
3 cups canned, crushed tomatoes
2 cups tomato sauce
⅓ cup roughly chopped basil
¼ cup roughly chopped Italian parsley
½ teaspoon crushed red pepper
2 teaspoons salt

13-15 ounces gluten-free lasagna sheets
1½–2 cups lemon-herb cashew ricotta (page 112)
Fresh minced basil, to top

1. In a Dutch oven or large skillet, sauté the onions on medium-high heat in olive oil until translucent. Add in the ground beef, breaking it apart as it cooks down. Once the beef starts to brown, add in the garlic, crushed tomatoes, tomato sauce, basil, parsley, crushed red pepper, and salt. Reduce the heat to low, cover the pot, and allow the sauce to simmer on low for at least 30 minutes and up to 4 hours, stirring every so often (see note below).

2. Once the meat sauce is done simmering, preheat the oven to 375 degrees. Fill a large pot with water and bring it to a boil. Par-boil the lasagna noodles 2–3 minutes just until they are flexible (do not fully cook the noodles or they will turn to mush in the oven). In a medium-large sized casserole dish, first spread a thin layer of meat sauce, top with 3–4 lasagna sheets, top the lasagna sheets with a layer of the lemon-herb cashew ricotta, and then meat sauce. Continue layering this way until you have at least 3 layers (the top layer being the meat sauce).

3. Cover the casserole dish with foil and bake for 40–45 minutes, then remove the foil and bake 10 minutes more. Allow the lasagna to cool a few minutes once out of the oven. Slice the lasagna and serve topped with fresh basil.

> **NOTE:** I really recommended making your meat sauce as early in the day as possible, if you have the time. Allowing the meat sauce to simmer on low for a few hours really develops the flavors of the sauce and you end up with a richer tasting dish.

SHRIMP PAD THAI

Gluten-Free, Dairy-Free

2–3 Servings

One of my fondest memories is when Jason and I were dating and he introduced me to Thai food for the first time. The first Thai dish I ever tried was Shrimp Pad Thai, and I must say, to this day it's still my favorite. Pad Thai is traditionally made with rice noodles in a sweet and tangy sauce with ingredients like bean sprouts, egg, crushed peanuts, and lime juice. As strange as the combinations of ingredients may seem, they somehow work beautifully together and you end up with a fabulous-tasting noodle dish.

Pad-Thai Sauce:
¼ cup lime juice
¼ cup coconut aminos
2 tablespoons honey
1 tablespoon coconut oil
¼ teaspoon crushed red pepper

6 ounces brown rice pad-Thai noodles
10 large shrimp, peeled and de-veined
2 tablespoons coconut oil
2 garlic cloves, minced
1 teaspoon ginger, grated
1 cup green onions, roughly chopped
2 eggs, whisked

Serve with:
1 cup mung bean sprouts
½ cup cilantro, roughly chopped
Crushed peanuts, as desired
Plenty of lime wedges
Chili sauce, as desired

1. In a bowl, mix together all sauce ingredients and set aside.

2. Fill a large bowl with warm water and soak the pad Thai noodles 10–15 minutes, or as directed on the package.

3. In a large skillet or wok, sauté the shrimp in 1 tablespoon of coconut oil with the garlic, ginger, and green onions for a few minutes until the shrimp is pink and cooked. Remove from the skillet and set aside. Add the whisked eggs to the same skillet and sauté until cooked. Remove the eggs from the skillet and set aside.

4. Turn the heat up on the skillet and add 1 tablespoon of coconut oil. Drain the soaked rice noodles (they should feel soft, not firm) and add the rice noodles to the hot skillet, frying them in the oil about 30 seconds. Now add the shrimp mixture, eggs, and Pad Thai sauce to the skillet and combine everything well. Once the sauce is nearly absorbed, turn the heat off and transfer the noodles to a large plate. Top the pad-Thai with the mung bean sprouts, cilantro, crushed peanuts, and drizzle the noodles with plenty of lime juice. Serve with chili sauce for added heat.

> **NOTE:** Traditional Pad Thai recipes use fish sauce and Tamarind paste. Fish sauce has an incredibly high amount of sodium (1 tablespoon equaling nearly 1,400 mg of sodium!), so I replaced it with coconut aminos. Tamarind paste can be hard to find in stores, so to make this recipe a bit less complicated I use lime juice instead.

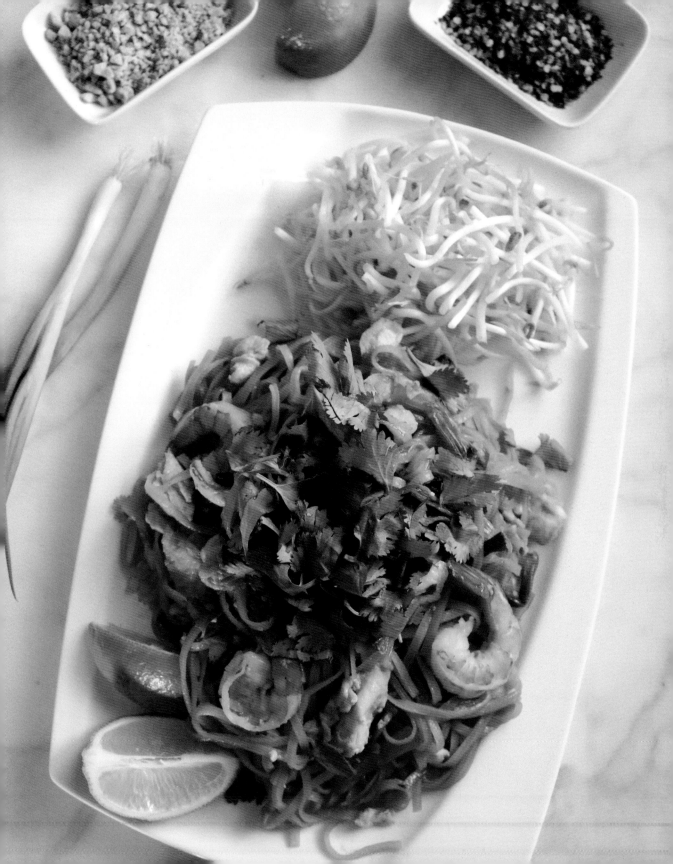

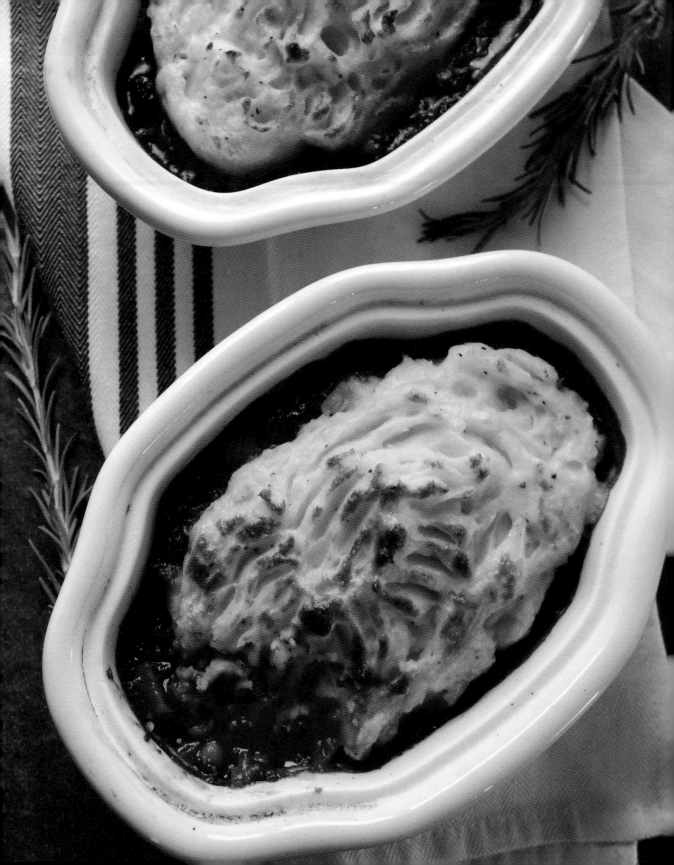

SHEPHERD'S PIE

Gluten-Free, Dairy-Free
4 Servings

Shepherd's pie makes me want to cozy up with a blanket next to a warm fire and watch the rain fall outside. This is a dish with a layer of cooked meat and vegetables topped with mashed potatoes, baked until the potatoes are well-browned. I love to make this recipe in individual ramekin dishes for a marvelous presentation.

Meat Filling:

1 cup minced yellow onions
2 tablespoons extra-virgin olive oil
1 pound ground beef
½ pound cubed lamb (optional)
4 garlic cloves, minced
2 tablespoons gluten-free flour
2 tablespoons tomato paste
2 cups low-sodium beef broth
1 cup diced carrots
1 tablespoon Worcestershire sauce
2 teaspoons minced rosemary
1 teaspoon minced thyme
1 teaspoon paprika
1½ teaspoons salt
½ teaspoon pepper
½ cup cooked peas

Mashed Potato Topping:

1 pound russet potatoes, peeled
1¼ cup full-fat coconut milk
1 teaspoon salt
1 teaspoon garlic powder
½ teaspoon black pepper
1 egg yolk, whisked

1. Preheat your oven to 375 degrees.

2. In a large skillet or Dutch oven, sauté the onions in olive oil on medium-high heat until translucent. Add in the ground beef, breaking it apart with a spatula. Once the beef is browned, add in the lamb and garlic, sautéing everything for 1–2 minutes. Sprinkle the flour over the mixture then add in tomato paste, combining everything together well. Add in the broth, carrots, Worcestershire sauce, rosemary, thyme, paprika, salt, and pepper. Bring everything to a boil then reduce the heat to low, cover the pot, and let simmer at least 30 minutes, stirring every so often. Once the filling is done simmering, add in the peas.

3. While the filling is simmering, boil your potatoes in a large pot of water for 20 minutes or until they are cooked through and fork tender. Drain and place in a large bowl. Mash the potatoes down then add in the coconut milk and spices. Mix the potatoes until completely smooth and no chunks are visible. Once cooled, transfer to a large plastic bag and cut the bottom tip off the bag.

4. Assemble a medium casserole dish (or four individual-sized ramekins), and spoon the meat filling evenly. Pipe the mashed potatoes through the plastic bag on top of the filling. Use a fork to create nice peaks in the mashed potatoes. Brush the tops of the mashed potatoes gently with the whisked egg yolk.

> Bake for 15–20 minutes, then turn the oven to broil. Broil for 3–4 minutes or until the mashed potato peaks are browned. Remove from the oven and serve immediately.

SLOPPY JOE STUFFED BAKED POTATOES

Gluten-Free, Dairy-Free, Grain-Free

4 Servings

Ditch the store-bought, processed, and chemical-filled sloppy joe mixture for this homemade rendition. This sloppy joe sauce is so flavorful and hearty, and instead of making it into a sandwich, you stuff baked potatoes with it for a meaty, satisfying dinner.

Sloppy Joe Filling:

1 cup minced yellow onions
1 cup minced carrots
1 cup minced celery
4 garlic cloves, minced
2 tablespoons extra-virgin olive oil
1 pound ground beef
1 cup canned tomato sauce
3 tablespoons tomato paste
¼ cup minced Italian parsley
2 tablespoons Worcestershire
*   sauce*
1 tablespoon + 1 teaspoon honey
1 teaspoon paprika
1 teaspoon chili powder
½ teaspoon salt
½ teaspoon crushed red pepper

4 medium-sized russet potatoes
Salt and black pepper, as desired
Fresh minced chives, to top

1. Preheat the oven to 400 degrees. Poke holes on the tops of the baked potatoes and place them directly on the oven rack. Bake the potatoes for 45–60 minutes or until they are cooked through.

2. In a large skillet, sauté the onions, carrots, celery, and garlic on medium-high heat in the olive oil about 5 minutes. Add in the ground beef, breaking it apart with a spatula. Once the beef is nearly cooked and browned, add in the tomato sauce, tomato paste, parsley, Worcestershire sauce, honey, paprika, chili powder, salt, and crushed red pepper, combining all ingredients together well. Reduce the heat to low, cover the skillet, and let the filling simmer at least 30 minutes, or while the potatoes finish cooking.

3. Remove the baked potatoes from the oven once cooked then slice ¼ of the top off the baked potato. Gently scoop out some of the inside of the potato, then sprinkle the tops with salt and black pepper. Generously stuff each potato with the sloppy joe filling and top with fresh chives. Serve immediately.

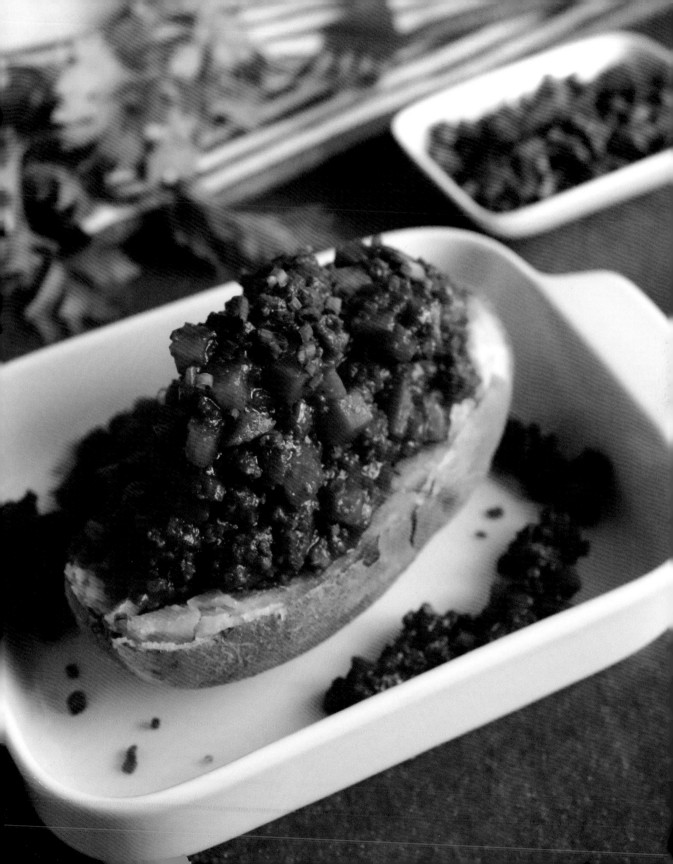

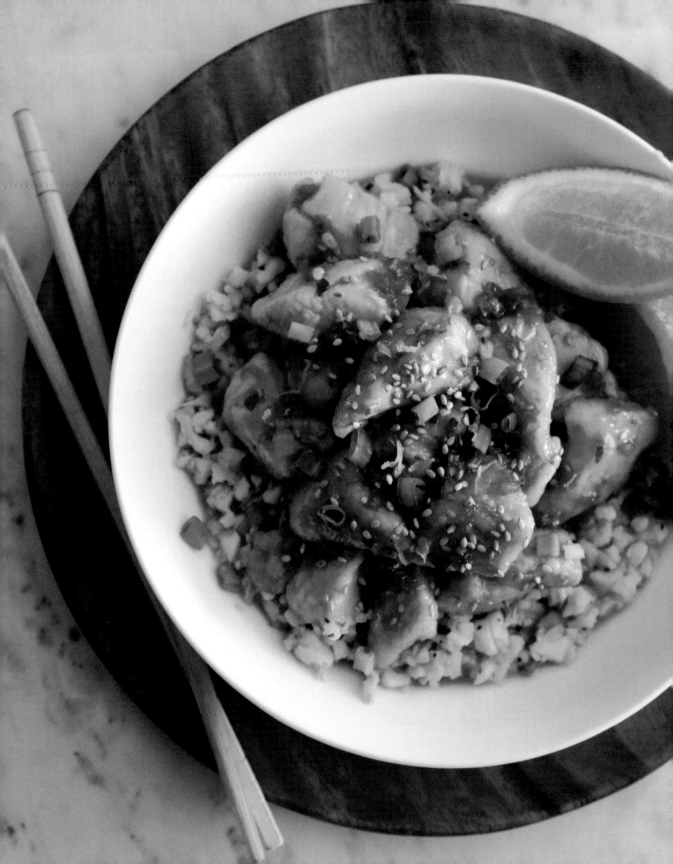

ORANGE CHICKEN

Gluten-Free, Dairy-Free

2 Servings

One of my favorite pastimes is ordering orange chicken from a local fast food Chinese restaurant. Unfortunately, traditional orange chicken is packed with unhealthy ingredients, so I created an easy, at-home version that has all-natural ingredients and tastes amazing to boot.

1 pound chicken breasts, cubed
2 tablespoons gluten-free flour
2 tablespoons avocado oil

Orange Sauce:
4 garlic cloves, minced
1 tablespoon grated ginger
2 teaspoons sesame oil
1¼ cups fresh-squeezed orange juice
1 tablespoon orange zest
¼ cup honey
3 tablespoons coconut aminos
½ teaspoon crushed red pepper

Toppings:
Green onions, diced
Sesame seeds
Sriracha sauce, for added spice

Serve with cauliflower rice or brown rice

1. In a small saucepan, sauté the garlic and ginger in the sesame oil about 30 seconds. Then add in the orange juice, zest, honey, coconut aminos, and crushed red pepper. Bring the sauce to a rapid boil, whisking it constantly. Reduce the heat to medium, and allow the sauce to reduce and thicken about 30 minutes, stirring it every so often.

2. Place the cubed chicken in a large plastic bag with the flour and shake it until the chicken is completely covered. Heat up the avocado oil in a skillet and add in the floured chicken pieces. Fry each side of the chicken for 2–3 minutes. Pour the orange sauce all over the chicken, and let it simmer in the sauce a few more minutes or until cooked through.

3. Serve the orange chicken over cauliflower rice or brown rice topped with green onions, sesame seeds, and sriracha sauce.

LEMON-CREAM SPAGHETTI SQUASH WITH CHICKEN SAUSAGE

Gluten-Free, Dairy-Free

3–4 Servings

One of our best-loved dishes is this lemon-cream pasta from a little Italian restaurant by our house. Unfortunately, that lemon-cream sauce is loaded with dairy, so I came up with a lightened-up, dairy-free version that is equally as satisfying.

3–4 pounds of spaghetti squash
2 tablespoons extra-virgin olive oil
6 ounces chicken sausage, sliced
12 asparagus spears, cut in thirds

Lemon-Cream Sauce:
2 tablespoons gluten-free flour
2 tablespoons extra-virgin olive oil
2 cups unsweetened almond milk, warmed
2 tablespoons lemon juice
1 teaspoon lemon zest
1 tablespoon honey
1 teaspoon garlic powder
1 teaspoon salt
1 teaspoon black pepper
½ teaspoon crushed red pepper

1. Preheat your oven to 400 degrees. Cut the spaghetti squash in half, then scoop out the seeds. Brush the top of the spaghetti squash in 1 tablespoon of olive oil then place on a baking sheet face-down. Bake for 45–60 minutes, depending on the size of the squash.

2. In a saucepan, start by making a roux with the 2 tablespoons flour and 2 tablespoons olive oil. Once a paste is formed after a few seconds, slowly add in the warmed almond milk, whisking it constantly until the sauce thickens. Once the sauce has thickened, add in the lemon juice, zest, honey, garlic powder, salt, black pepper, and crushed red pepper, and combine all ingredients well. Reduce the heat to low and let the sauce simmer until a desired thickness has been attained.

3. In a large skillet, cook the chicken sausage and asparagus in 1 tablespoon of olive oil for a few minutes or until the chicken is cooked through.

4. Remove the spaghetti squash from the oven and allow it to cool. Using a fork, gently scoop out the squash from the skin. Add the spaghetti squash to the skillet with the chicken sausage and asparagus, then pour the lemon cream sauce over it. Mix everything together well and serve immediately.

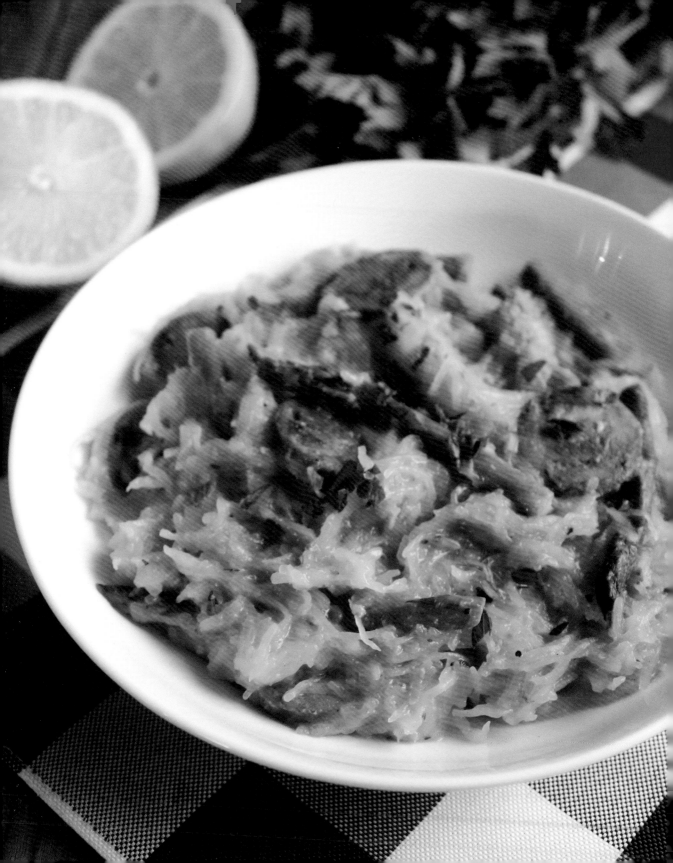

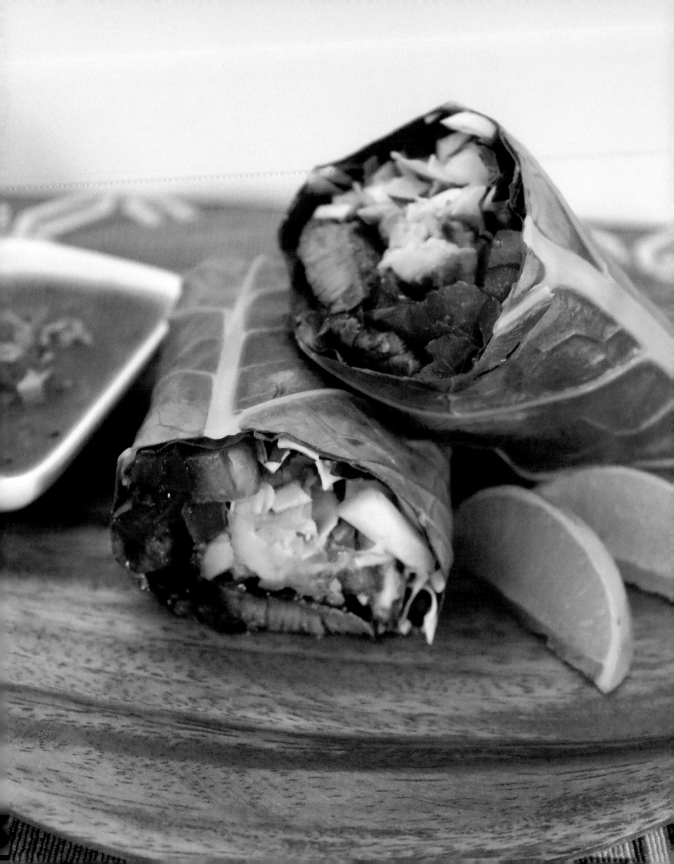

STEAK FAJITA COLLARD-WRAPPED BURRITOS

Gluten-Free, Dairy-Free, Grain-Free

Serves 2

Jason always said the thing he misses most since going gluten-free is burritos, so I made him these collard-wrapped burritos one day, and he loved them! Collard greens are a large-leafed vegetable and are the perfect replacement for tortillas because of their flexibility and durability. Stuffing them with this fajita mixture makes you feel like you're eating a real burrito at your favorite Mexican restaurant!

4 large collard green leaves
1 small onion, sliced thin
1 red bell pepper, sliced thin
2 tablespoons extra-virgin olive oil
½ pound steak (such as rib eye),
    sliced into strips
½ teaspoon salt
¼ teaspoon black pepper
½ teaspoon chili powder
½ teaspoon cumin

Toppings:

½ cup diced tomatoes
1 avocado, pitted and smashed
1 cup shredded green cabbage
1 tablespoon minced cilantro

Serve with fresh salsa

> **TIP:** Try and find the largest collard greens leaves as possible. It's easier to roll the burritos!

1. Fill a large frying pan ¾ of the way with water. Bring the water to a boil. On a cutting board, take each collard green leaf and using a sharp knife, shave the thick stalk down until it is the same thickness as the leaf. This will allow the leaf to become more flexible for wrapping.

2. Using a pair of tongs, place each collard leaf (one at a time) into the boiling water for about 30 seconds. Remove the collard leaf and lightly pat the excess water off with a paper towel.

3. In a pan, sauté your onions and bell peppers in the olive oil a few minutes or until they are nicely browned. Add in the sliced steak, salt, pepper, chili powder, and cumin, then sauté for 2–4 minutes depending on how you prefer your steak to be prepared.

4. To assemble the burritos: Lay out two collard green leaves on a cutting board, slightly overlapping each other. On the right side of the leaf, add in the steak fajita mixture, then top with the tomatoes, avocado, cabbage, and cilantro. You will roll this like a burrito, gently folding in the sides and wrapping it tight. Once the burrito is rolled, slice it in half. Serve with fresh salsa.

BUTTERNUT SQUASH MAC AND CHEESE

Gluten-Free, Dairy-Free, Vegan
3–4 Servings

Who doesn't love mac and cheese? This butternut squash cheese sauce could almost fool anyone—it tastes so cheesy! The blend of butternut squash with cashews and nutritional yeast makes this mac and cheese taste like the real deal. This recipe is incredibly simple to make and so tasty.

"Cheese Sauce:"
½ cup raw cashews
3 cups cubed butternut squash
1 cup thinly sliced yellow onions
5 garlic cloves, peeled and
   smashed
2 tablespoons extra-virgin olive oil
1 cup unsweetened almond milk
2 tablespoons nutritional yeast
   flakes
1 teaspoon mustard powder
¼ teaspoon paprika
1 teaspoon salt

Bread Crumbs:
⅓ cup gluten-free panko bread
   crumbs
2 teaspoons extra-virgin olive oil
Pinch of salt

8–10 ounces gluten-free elbow
   macaroni noodles
Minced parsley, to top

Serve with a side of sriracha sauce
   (page 128)

1. Soak the cashews in a bowl with water for 30 minutes. Boil the butternut squash in water about 10 minutes, or until fork tender. While the squash is boiling, sauté the onions and garlic in 2 tablespoons of olive oil until the onions are translucent.

2. Drain the squash from the water and transfer it to a blender along with the sautéed garlic cloves, onions, soaked cashews, and almond milk. Blend on high until the sauce is completely smooth. Transfer the sauce into a Dutch oven or large skillet and turn the heat to low. Now add in the nutritional yeast, mustard powder, paprika, and salt. Cover the pan and simmer the sauce on low heat.

3. Combine the bread crumbs, 2 teaspoons of olive oil, and salt in a skillet on medium-high heat and stir the bread crumbs around for 3 minutes, or until they are toasted and nicely browned. Remove the bread crumbs from the heat and set aside.

4. Cook your elbow macaroni noodles according to the package. Once the noodles are al dente, drain them then add them to the butternut squash sauce. Combine the noodles with the sauce until all noodles are covered. Serve the butternut squash mac and cheese topped with the breadcrumbs and minced parsley.

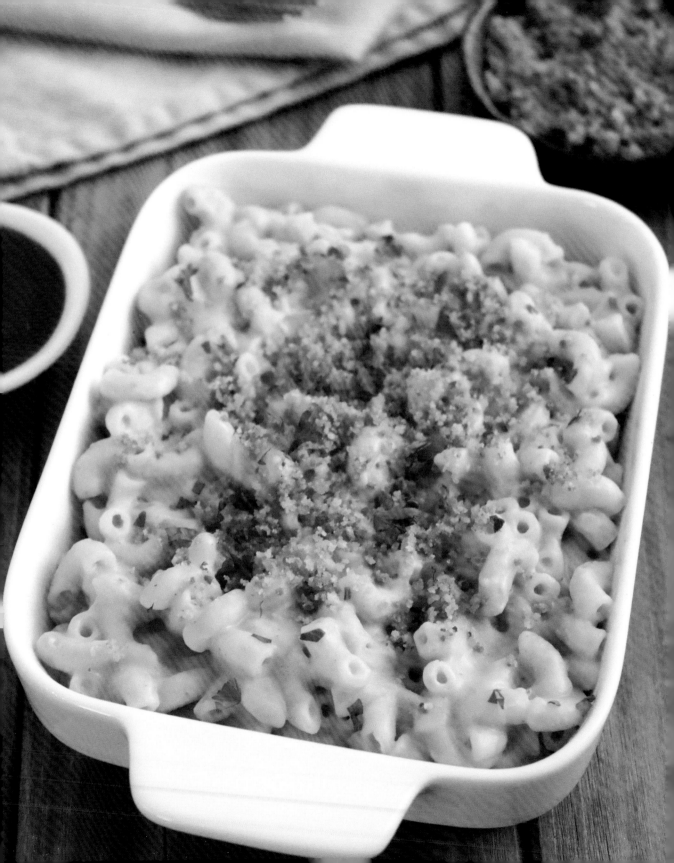

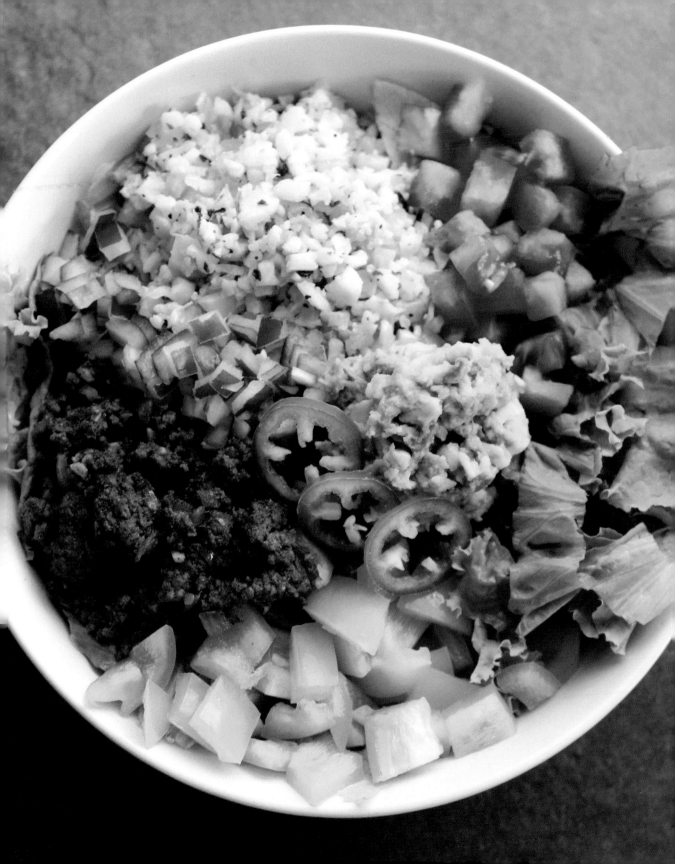

DECONSTRUCTED BURRITO BOWLS WITH CILANTRO-LIME CAULIFLOWER RICE

Gluten-Free, Dairy-Free, Grain-Free

2–3 Servings

Inspired by Chipotle's bowls, this deconstructed burrito bowl is everything you want out of a meal. The taco meat is so flavor-packed and the cilantro-lime cauliflower rice is fantastic. I make these bowls all the time for dinner and they never disappoint.

Taco Meat:
½ cup minced yellow onions
1 tablespoon extra-virgin olive oil
½ pound ground beef
4 garlic cloves, minced
1 teaspoon paprika
1 teaspoon chili powder
1½ teaspoons cumin
½ teaspoon black pepper
½ teaspoon salt

Cilantro-Lime Cauliflower Rice:
½ cup minced yellow onions
2 tablespoons extra-virgin olive oil
2½ cups riced cauliflower
2 garlic cloves, minced
2 tablespoons lime juice
⅓ cup minced cilantro
½ teaspoon salt
½ teaspoon black pepper

4 cups shredded green leaf lettuce
¼ cup minced red onions
1 large avocado, smashed
½ cup diced tomatoes
1 cup chopped yellow bell pepper
Jalapeño slices, as desired

Serve with fresh salsa

1. For the taco meat, in a skillet, sauté the onions on medium-high heat in 1 tablespoon of olive oil until translucent. Add in the beef and garlic, breaking up the beef with a spatula until crumbled. Once the beef is nearly cooked, season it with the paprika, chili powder, cumin, pepper, and salt. Turn the heat to low and let the beef simmer on low heat.

2. For the rice, in a separate skillet, sauté the onions in 2 tablespoons of olive oil until translucent. Add in the riced cauliflower and garlic. Sauté on medium heat for about 5 minutes. Then add in the lime juice, cilantro, salt, and pepper. You want the cauliflower rice to be cooked, but still firm.

3. To assemble the bowls, place the shredded lettuce at the bottom of a bowl then top it with the ground beef, cauliflower rice, red onions, avocado, tomatoes, bell peppers, and jalapeño slices. Serve the burrito bowls with fresh salsa.

TIP: You can buy organic pre-packaged cauliflower rice at Trader Joe's! You can also make cauliflower rice at home by placing the cauliflower florets in a food processor and pulsing the floret's until they have a rice-like consistency.

SHRIMP AND KALE FETTUCINE IN A CAULIFLOWER CREAM SAUCE

Gluten-Free, Dairy-Free

4 Servings

I'm obsessed with this cauliflower cream sauce. It tastes so similar to an alfredo sauce, it's insane. Every time I make this sauce, I find myself eating it by the spoonful—it's that good! The sauce is perfectly complemented by the shrimp, bacon, and kale with fettuccine noodles for a delightful, yet simple dinner.

Cauliflower Cream Sauce:

1 medium-sized head of cauliflower, roughly chopped
1 large sweet onion, minced
5 garlic cloves, minced
2 tablespoons extra-virgin olive oil
2 cups unsweetened almond milk
1 teaspoon salt
½ teaspoon black pepper
¼ teaspoon crushed red pepper

4 slices all-natural bacon, diced
2 cups packed kale, roughly chopped
½ pound wild caught shrimp, peeled and deveined
½ teaspoon salt
½ teaspoon black pepper
About 10 ounces gluten-free fettuccine noodles
Fresh minced parsley, to top

1. Boil the cauliflower in a large pot of water about 5–8 minutes or until fork tender. Drain the cauliflower from the water and transfer it to a blender. While the cauliflower is boiling, in a skillet sauté the onions and garlic in 2 tablespoons of olive oil until the onions are translucent. Add the sautéed onions and garlic to the blender along with the almond milk, salt, and peppers. Blend on high until the sauce is completely smooth. Transfer the sauce to a Dutch oven or large skillet and let it simmer on low heat.

2. In a skillet, cook your diced bacon pieces until they are crispy, then remove from the pan and set it aside, rendering the bacon fat. Add the kale and shrimp to the skillet and sauté for 4–5 minutes or until the shrimp is cooked. Season the shrimp and kale with salt and pepper. Remove from heat and set aside.

3. Cook your fettuccine noodles according to the package. Once the noodles are cooked al dente, drain them then add the noodles into the cauliflower cream sauce. Add the shrimp, kale, and bacon in with the noodles and sauce and toss the pasta together. Serve immediately topped with minced parsley.

> **FACT:** Kale is one of the most nutrient-dense foods in the world because of its low calorie content and high nutrient density. It's packed full of fiber and vitamins such as iron, Vitamin K, and magnesium. Kale actually has more iron per calorie than beef!

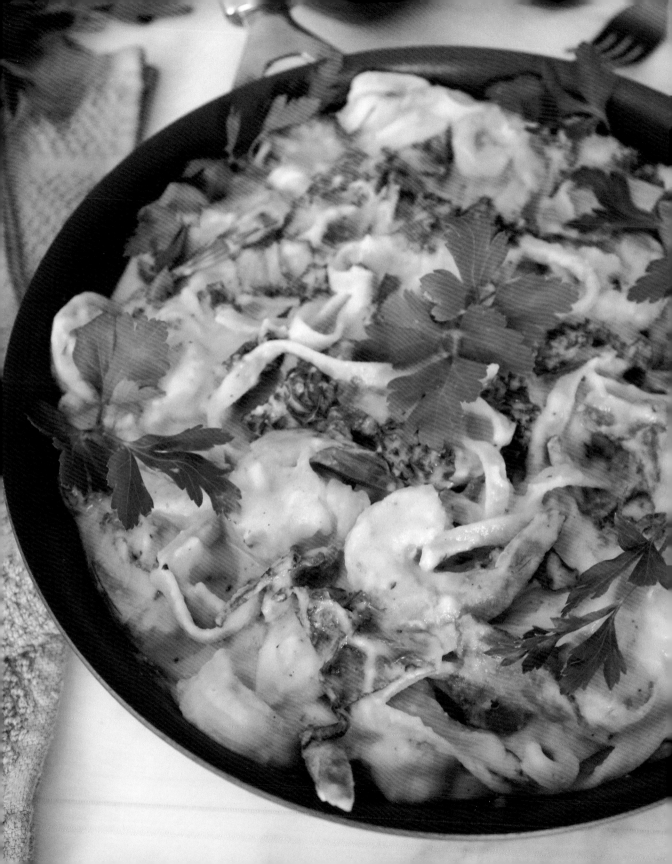

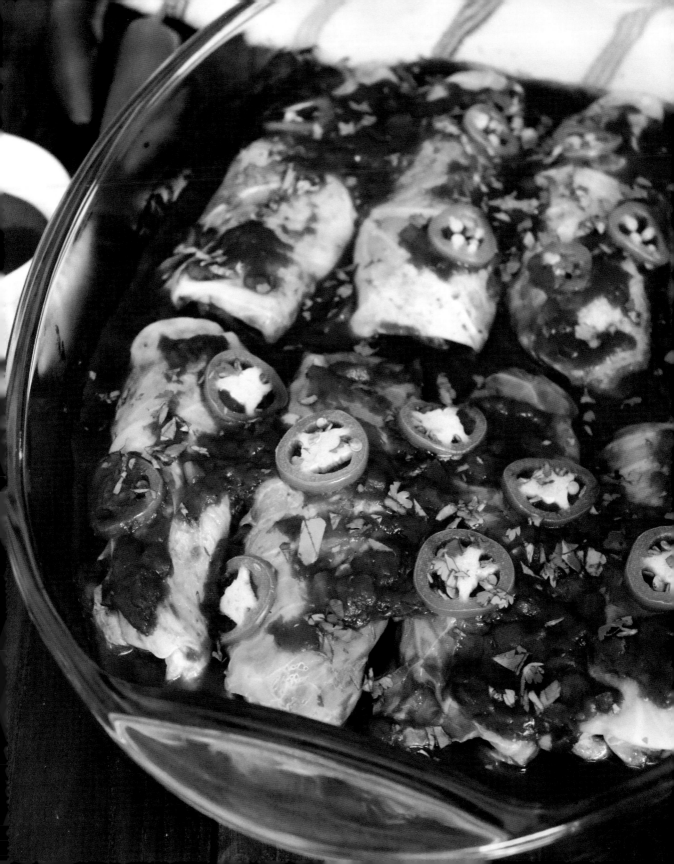

JALAPEÑO-BARBEQUE STUFFED CABBAGE ROLLS

Gluten-Free, Dairy-Free

Serves 3–4 (Makes about 8 rolls)

Cabbage rolls are cooked cabbage leaves stuffed with a meat filling, then rolled and baked. I put a twist on traditional cabbage rolls by adding a sweet barbeque sauce and kicking up the heat with jalapeños. This hearty dish is perfect for cold winter months when you feel like some healthy comfort food.

Sauce:

½ yellow onion, minced
4 garlic cloves, minced
½ jalapeño, minced
2 tablespoons extra-virgin olive oil
15 ounce can tomato sauce or
    tomato puree
½ cup barbeque sauce
½ teaspoon salt
½ teaspoon black pepper

Filling:

½ yellow onion, minced
4 garlic cloves, minced
½ jalapeño, minced
1 tablespoon extra-virgin olive oil
1 pound ground beef
1 cup cooked brown rice
3 tablespoons barbeque sauce
⅓ cup minced cilantro
1 teaspoon paprika
½ teaspoon salt
½ teaspoon black pepper

1 large head green cabbage
1 small jalapeño, sliced thin
Cilantro minced, to top

1. Preheat your oven to 375 degrees.

2. Fill a large pot with water and bring it to a boil. Using a knife, gently cut the core out of the cabbage head. Place the whole cabbage head in the boiling water about 5 minutes or until the outer leaves are softened. Remove as many leaves as possible, then for the inner leaves that aren't cooked as well, return them to the boiling water until softened. Pat the cabbage leaves dry and set aside.

3. In a saucepan, sauté the onions, garlic, and jalapeños in olive oil until the onions are translucent. Add in the tomato sauce, barbeque sauce, and seasonings. Bring the sauce to a boil then reduce the heat to low and allow the sauce to simmer while you prepare the filling.

4. In a skillet, sauté the onions, garlic, and jalapeños in olive oil until the onions are translucent. Add in the ground beef, breaking it down with a spatula. Once the beef is cooked, add in the cooked rice, barbeque sauce, cilantro, and seasonings. Transfer to a large bowl.

5. To assemble the cabbage rolls, first spread a thin layer of your sauce in a casserole dish. Scoop a generous amount of filling into each cabbage leaf then roll it like an egg roll, tucking in the ends. Place each cabbage roll in the casserole dish. Pour the rest of the sauce over the cabbage rolls then top them with a layer of thinly sliced jalapeños. Cover the casserole dish with foil and bake for 40–45 minutes. Remove the cabbage rolls from the oven and serve topped with fresh cilantro.

Resource List

This is a list of material that helped me when I initially started researching the healing benefits of food, going organic, avoiding GMOs, and eating a gluten- and dairy-free diet. I hope some of these resources will help you in your journey to health and wellness, just as they helped Jason and I.

Informative Websites:
EWG.org
Nongmoproject.org
Foodfacts.com
Foodbabe.com
Organicconsumers.org
Livingmaxwell.com

Documentaries:
GMO OMG
Food, Inc.
The Future of Food
Food Matters
Super Size Me

Books:
The Gluten Connection: How Gluten Sensitivity May Be Sabotaging Your Health—And What You Can Do to Take Control Now—by Shari Lieberman

Organic Manifesto: How Organic Food Can Heal Our Planet, Feed the World, and Keep Us Safe—by Maria Rodale

Gluten Freedom: The Nation's Leading Expert Offers the Essential Guide to a Healthy, Gluten-Free Lifestyle—by Alessio Fasano, Susie Flaherty

Whitewash: The Disturbing Truth About Cow's Milk and Your Health—by Joseph Keon

Acknowledgments

Jason:

You are my rock and I would be completely lost without you. I am so grateful to have gone through this journey of life with you by my side. Thank you for being my number-one recipe critic, making me laugh even in the darkest of times, and never letting me forget who my best friend and partner in life is.

Family and Friends:

Thank you for always being there by our side through the best and the worst of times, and for giving us your endless love, patience, and support. You know who each of you are and we love you all so dearly.

Jim and Laura LaValle:

You changed the way we view food forever, and ultimately saved Jason's life. We are forever grateful to you both.

Vicki Marsdon and Wordlink Literary Agency:

Thank you for believing in me and taking the time to read my proposal. You saw my vision from the very beginning, and this cookbook would not be here if it weren't for you.

My Book Editor, Leah Zarra:

Thank you for putting up with all my silly, first-time author questions and helping guide me through the process of creating a book. I will be forever grateful for your patience and kindness.

Skyhorse Publishing:

Thank you for taking a chance on a first-time author and making my dreams of having a published cookbook a reality.

Photography:

Thank you to Sub Zero and Wolf Showroom Costa Mesa, CA for allowing me to use your beautiful demo kitchen for my pictures.

Thank you to Amanda Allphin Photography for taking such lovely photos of Jason and I. You are such a talented photographer and a true visionary.

Followers:

Thank you to the readers of my blog and my followers on Instagram. The times when I wanted to give up, you guys were always there to inspire me to keep going and never give up on my dream. It brings me so much pleasure to create recipes and in turn see people re-make my recipes around the world. That will always and forever be a pinch-me moment.

Recipe Index

Conversion Charts

METRIC AND IMPERIAL CONVERSIONS
(These conversions are rounded for convenience)

Ingredient	Cups/Tablespoons/Teaspoons	Ounces	Grams/Milliliters
Butter	1 cup/ 16 tablespoons/ 2 sticks	8 ounces	230 grams
Cheese, shredded	1 cup	4 ounces	110 grams
Cream cheese	1 tablespoon	0.5 ounce	14.5 grams
Cornstarch	1 tablespoon	0.3 ounce	8 grams
Flour, all-purpose	1 cup/1 tablespoon	4.5 ounces/0.3 ounce	125 grams/8 grams
Flour, whole wheat	1 cup	4 ounces	120 grams
Fruit, dried	1 cup	4 ounces	120 grams
Fruits or veggies, chopped	1 cup	5 to 7 ounces	145 to 200 grams
Fruits or veggies, puréed	1 cup	8.5 ounces	245 grams
Honey, maple syrup, or corn syrup	1 tablespoon	0.75 ounce	20 grams
Liquids: cream, milk, water, or juice	1 cup	8 fluid ounces	240 milliliters
Oats	1 cup	5.5 ounces	150 grams
Salt	1 teaspoon	0.2 ounces	6 grams
Spices: cinnamon, cloves, ginger, or nutmeg (ground)	1 teaspoon	0.2 ounce	5 milliliters
Sugar, brown, firmly packed	1 cup	7 ounces	200 grams
Sugar, white	1 cup/1 tablespoon	7 ounces/0.5 ounce	200 grams/12.5 grams
Vanilla extract	1 teaspoon	0.2 ounce	4 grams

OVEN TEMPERATURES

Fahrenheit	Celsius	Gas Mark
225°	110°	¼
250°	120°	½
275°	140°	1
300°	150°	2
325°	160°	3
350°	180°	4
375°	190°	5
400°	200°	6
425°	220°	7
450°	230°	8